Elisabeth von der Lohe

Coronary Heart Disease in Women

D0733454

Springer

Berlin
Heidelberg
New York
Hong Kong
London
Milan
Paris
Tokyo

Elisabeth von der Lohe

Coronary Heart Disease in Women

Prevention · Diagnosis · Therapy

With 37 Figures and 34 Tables

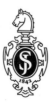 Springer

Elisabeth von der Lohe MD

Associate Professor of Clinical Medicine (Cardiology)
Chief of Cardiology, Wishard Health Services
Krannert Institute of Cardiology, Indiana University
Clarian Cardiovascular Center
1800 N Senate Blvd B 400
Indianapolis, IN 46202, USA
e-mail: evonderl@iupui.edu

ISBN 3-540-00128-X Springer-Verlag Berlin Heidelberg New York

Cataloging-in-Publication Data applied for
Bibliographic information published by Die Deutsche Bibliothek
Die Deutsche Bibliothek lists this publication in the Deutsche Nationalbibliografie;
detailed bibliographic data is available in the Internet at <http://dnb.ddb.de>.

Springer-Verlag Berlin Heidelberg New York
a member of BertelsmannSpringer Science + Business Media GmbH
http://www.springer.de
© Springer-Verlag Berlin Heidelberg 2003
Printed in Germany

Production: PRO EDIT GmbH, 69126 Heidelberg, Germany
Cover design: deblik, Berlin, Germany
Typesetting and Repro: AM-productions GmbH, 69168 Wiesloch, Germany
Printed on acid-free paper   21/3135Re – 5 4 3 2 1 0

Foreword

Until recently coronary artery disease was thought to be primarily a disease in men. This misconception has led to a great deal of misunderstanding and mismanagement of women who have coronary heart disease. We now know that coronary heart disease is a major problem in women. Not only is the frequency of coronary artery disease in women higher than previously recognized, but in women this disease also has some unique management differences that must be understood. This book is appropriate, timely, and necessary, as physicians are responsible for our increasingly aging population; thus, it is important to know the issues that relate to women and coronary heart disease. The differences between men and women in patients with coronary heart disease are quite numerous and profound.

Dr. von der Lohe discusses these differences and the appropriate management in depth. Our knowledge is changing rapidly, and it is essential for clinicians to be kept up-to-date as to how best to manage women who suffer from this problem. Dr. von der Lohe is a very appropriate person to address this issue since she not only runs a women's health clinic, but also is actively involved in the most frequently used diagnostic and therapeutic efforts at managing coronary artery disease, namely, echocardiography and both diagnostic and interventional cardiac catheterization.

I am honored to have been asked to write this introduction. I am certain that this text will go a long way toward improving our understanding and management of women with coronary heart disease.

Harvey Feigenbaum
Distinguished Professor of Medicine
Director, Echocardiography Laboratories
Indiana University School of Medicine
Senior Research Associate
Indianapolis, Indiana, United States

Preface

Coronary artery disease has stereotypically been characterized as a men's disease.

The fact is, however, that as many women as men die from coronary artery disease each year in the United States. In women 75 years of age or older, it is even the leading cause of death. Women tend to be older at the time when the diagnosis of coronary artery disease is made, and, on average, a myocardial infarct strikes about 20 years later in women than in men. The increase in the incidence of coronary artery disease with age correlates with the decline in the serum estrogen levels in women entering menopause. Because many women now live 40 years or more beyond the onset of menopause, coronary artery disease in aging women will most certainly play a predominant role in future medicine. Not many physicians have realized its growing significance. Increasing awareness of these epidemiological changes will help improve health care for women with coronary artery diease.

Basic research over the past two decades or so has revealed fundamental differences in cardiovascular physiology between men and women. These findings led to the introduction of gender-specific approaches to diagnosis and treatment of coronary artery disease in clinical practice, and also caused an increase in the percentage of women that are included in clinical studies. Whereas 4 years ago only one quarter of study participants were females, this number has now risen to approximately 40 % and will most likely reach the 50 % mark over the course of the next decade. In the meantime, more and more programs for Women's Health have been established throughout the United States, specializing in prevention, diagnosis, and treatment of coronary artery diease in women. As director of a Women's Health Program and practicing interventional cardiologist, I was repeatedly asked to give seminars on cardiovascular disease in women. Based on this experience and following a suggestion by Dr. Udo K. Lindner, former at Springer-Verlag, editorial director, I came up with this textbook, which summarizes gender-specific differences in prevention, diagnosis and therapy of coronary artery disease. Special emphasis was placed on giving an account of current strategies for prevention of coronary artery disease and on discussing the current controversies in hormone replacement therapy.

Elisabeth von der Lohe
Indianapolis, February 2003

Contents

1 Epidemiology

Introduction. 2

Definition 2
    Gender-Specific Mortality Rates 3
    Morbidity and Mortality with Respect to Age and Gender 4
    Perception. 6
    Mortality in Myocardial Infarction:
    Comparison Between Women and Men 6
    International Comparisons 7

**The "MONItoring Cardiovascular Disease"
Project of the WHO (WHO MONICA Project)** 10

2 Cardiovascular Risk Factors and the Development of Coronary Heart Disease in Women

Smoking 16

Dyslipidemia 17

Lipoprotein (a) 19

Diabetes Mellitus. 20

Insulin Resistance and Polycystic Ovary Syndrome 21

**Family History of Coronary Heart Disease
or Genetic Disposition** 23

Hypertension 23

Sedentary Lifestyle 23

Obesity 25

Homocysteine 26

High sensitivity C-reactive Protein 27

Risk Factors Unique to Women 28
Menopause 28
Oral Contraception 29

3 Pathophysiology of Coronary Heart Disease and the Effects of Estrogen

Basics 36
Plaque Formation and Significance of Plaques in CHD 36

Effects of Estrogen 38
Effect of Estrogen on Vascular Reactivity
and Endothelial Function 39
Effect of Estrogen on Lipid Metabolism 41
Antioxidative Effect of Estrogen 42
Effect of Estrogen on Inflammation 43
Effect of Estrogen on Hemostasis 43

4 Stable Angina

Definition and Pathophysiology of Angina Pectoris 48

Diagnosis Based on Symptoms 49
Prinzmetal's or Variant Angina 50
Syndrome X 51

Diagnostic Evaluation 52
Electrocardiogram 52

Stress Testing, Including Stress Echocardiography
and Nuclear Imaging. 52
  Determination of Pretest Probability for CHD 52
  Selection of Stress Test 53
  Stress ECG. 53
  Nuclear Imaging 55
  Stress Echocardiography 56
  Pharmacological Stress Tests. 58
Electron Beam Computed Tomography 61
Magnetic Resonance Imaging. 61
Diagnostic Cardiac Catheterization. 61
Gender Differences in the Use of Diagnostic Cardiac
Catheterizations and Percutaneous Coronary Intervention 62

Medical Management. 64

  Beta-blockers 64
  Nitrate. 66
  Calcium Channel Blockers. 66

Percutaneous Coronary Intervention for Stable Angina . . . 67

  Gender-Specific Success and Complication Rates
  for Balloon Angioplasty 69
  Gender-Specific Success and Complication Rates
  for Coronary Intervention with Stent Implantation 71
  Restenosis. 74
  Rotablator Therapy, Directional Coronary Atherectomy,
  Laser Therapy. 74
  Multivessel Coronary Intervention – When PCI?
  When Bypass Surgery?. 75

5 Acute Myocardial Infarction

**Progression from Stable Coronary Heart Disease
to Myocardial Infarction** 84

Epidemiology of Acute Myocardial Infarction. 85

Pathophysiology 87

Clinical Presentation
of Acute Myocardial Infarction 89

Silent Myocardial Infarction 89
Symptomatic Myocardial Infarction 90

Criteria for the Diagnosis of Acute Myocardial Infarction . . . 90

Clinical Presentation 90
Electrocardiogram 91
Serum Markers of Cardiac Damage 91
Creatine Kinase and the CK Isoenzyme CK-MB 91
Troponin T and I 92

Therapy 92

Revascularization 93
Thrombolytic Therapy 93
Primary Percutaneous Transluminal Coronary Angioplasty . . 94
Thrombolysis Versus Primary PTCA 96
Rescue PTCA after Thrombolysis
of Acute Myocardial Infarction 97
Medical Therapy of Acute Myocardial Infarction 98
Aspirin 99
Beta-blockers 99
Unfractionated Heparin 99
Calcium Channel Blockers 100
ACE Inhibitors 100
Nitrates 100

Complications 101

Prognosis 102

Mortality in Acute Myocardial Infarction
(With and Without Thrombolysis) 103
Mortality in the Pre-thrombolytic Era
(Mid-1960s to Early-1980s) 105
Mortality in the Thrombolytic Era (1980 to Present) 105

**Influence of Gender on the Referral
for Coronary Angiography in Patients
with Acute Myocardial Infarction** 107

6 Acute Coronary Syndromes

Non-ST-Elevation Myocardial Infarction/Unstable Angina . . 116

Definition 118

Presentation 118

Diagnosis 119

Therapy 120
  Medical Therapy 120
    Aspirin 120
    Unfractionated Heparin 121
    Low-Molecular-Weight Heparin 121
    Glycoprotein IIb/IIIa Receptor Antagonists 122
    Nitrates 127
    Beta-blocker 127
    Calcium Channel Blocker 127
  Interventional Therapy 127

7 Coronary Artery Bypass Surgery

Operative Mortality 134

Complications Associated with CABG 138

Long-Term Outcomes 139

Indication for CABG Surgery 140

Comparison of CABG with Multivessel Angioplasty 141

8 Primary and Secondary Prevention of Coronary Heart Disease

Class I Interventions 148

  Treatment of Hyperlipidemia 148
    Diet 149
    Medical Therapy of Dyslipidemia 151
    Primary Prevention Trials 151
    Primary Prevention with Estrogen 151
    Secondary Prevention Trials with Statins 152
    Secondary Prevention Trials with
    Medications Other Than Statins 154
  Treatment of Hypertension 155
  Aspirin 160
    Primary Prevention of CAD with Aspirin 160
    Secondary Prevention with Aspirin 160

Class II Interventions 161

  Physical Activity 161
    Primary Prevention Studies 162
    Secondary Prevention Studies 162
  Weight Reduction 164
  Alcohol 164

Class III Interventions 166

  Antioxidants 166
    Vitamins E and C 166
    Beta-carotene 168

9 Hormone Replacement Therapy

**Hormone Replacement Therapy
and Prevention of Coronary Heart Disease** 176

**Observational Studies for Primary
and Secondary Prevention** 177

Randomized Primary Prevention Trials 178

Randomized Secondary Prevention Trials 180

Clinical Implications of Hormone Replacement Therapy . . . 185

Combination Therapy 187
Risk of Breast Cancer with HRT. 187
Risk of Ovarian Cancer with HRT 190
Risk of Endometrial Cancer with HRT 190
Risk of Deep Vein Thrombosis and Thromboembolic Events . . 191
Estrogen and High Sensitivity C-reactive Protein 192

Biological Mechanisms of Hormone Replacement Therapy . 193

Lipids and Antioxidant Effects of Estrogen 193
Glucose Metabolism 194
Hemostasis 195
Vascular Reactivity 195
Impact on Markers of Inflammation 196
Selective Estrogen Receptor Modulators 196
Soy Protein 198

10 Future Directions

Epidemiology

Introduction 2

Definition 2

Mortality in Myocardial Infarction:
Comparison Between Women and Men 6

The "MONItoring CArdiovascular Disease" Project
of the WHO (WHO MONICA Project). 10

References 12

Introduction

Cardiovascular disease (CVD) is still *the* leading cause of death in the industrialized world. It is the leading cause of death among women as well, often obscured by the fact that men have higher CVD morbidity and mortality rates before age 75 years. Even in developing countries CVD is on the rise, ranking a close second behind lower respiratory infections. In 1995 15 million people died of CVD, which accounted for 30 % of all deaths worldwide and 50 % of all deaths in the Western world. Seven million deaths were due to coronary heart disease and 4.6 % due to cerebrovascular disease. Eighty percent of these deaths occurred in individuals age 65 years or older [World Health Organization (WHO) statistics].

Definition

The WHO defines coronary heart disease as an acute or chronically impaired performance of the heart caused by a reduction or complete interruption of myocardial blood supply resulting from atherosclerosis of the cardiac arteries. Atherosclerosis of the coronary arteries leads to plaque formation and stenosis. Rupture of an atherosclerotic plaque with subsequent thrombus formation causes a complete or partial occlusion of the vessel. These processes manifest clinically as angina pectoris, unstable angina, myocardial infarction, heart failure, arrhythmia, and sudden cardiac death.

Although the definition of coronary heart disease (CHD) is the same worldwide, individual countries use different coding systems for the disease. This has a significant impact on the determination of the cause of death and consequently on death statistics. Most statistics are based on mortality data that are questionable for numerous reasons. In addition, a large number of women actually die from sudden cardiac death before being admitted to the hospital, and no confirmation of diagnosis occurs.

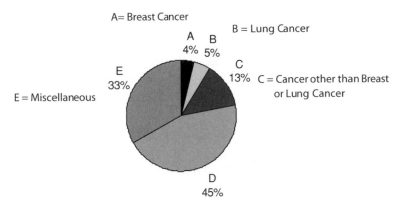

Fig. 1.1. Etiologies of mortality in women in the United States (WHO Statistics 1997)

Gender-Specific Mortality Rates

Cardiovascular disease is *the* leading cause of death in women in the United States. Approximately 50 % of all deaths are due to CVD, in particular due to CHD and stroke. Deaths due to CVD exceed the number of deaths from all cancers combined (Fig. 1.1).

In 1997 approximately 500,000 women died of CVD in the United States as opposed to 447,000 men. Among American women, 132,000 of the 500,000 deaths were due to ischemic heart disease and 97,000 due to myocardial infarction. These data far exceed the number of deaths from malignancies. In contrast to 500,000 deaths caused by CVD among women, only 42,000 were caused by breast cancer – the malignancy most feared by women. A total of 8700 women had fatal lung cancer, and 2000 died from cancer of the uterus. Over the course of her lifetime, a woman faces a 31 % probability to die from CHD and resulting illnesses. The risk of breast cancer is 2.8 %.

Morbidity and Mortality with Respect to Age and Gender

There is a significant difference in the incidence of CHD in women as compared with men. Independent of age, CHD occurs less frequently in women than in men; however, with increasing age this "advantage" gradually decreases. According to WHO statistics from 1997, 364 per 100,000 men 65–74 years of age died of CHD but only 168 per 100,000 women of the same age; however, after age 75 years cardiovascular mortality rates increase by a factor of 5 in men but by a factor of 9 in women. The fact that the absolute number of women dying from CVD is higher than that of men can be explained by the fact that a woman's average life expectancy is approximately 7–8 years higher than that of men, and that with increasing age the percentage of women within the general population increases as well. Up to the eighth decade the mortality rate by age is lower for women in every age group, but after age 70 years this ratio is reversed; thus, according to the WHO statistics for 1997, 31,000 men between 45–55 years died from cardiovascular diseases but only 13,000 women in the same age group. In the age group 65–75 years, the numbers were 104,000 men and 71,000 women; however, after age 75 years, the death rate from CVD was 243,000 for men and 382,000 for women (Table 1.1).

Numerous studies over the past 30 years primarily conducted in middle-aged men have led to the misconception that CHD is a men's disease. While it is true that the overall death rate caused by coronary artery disease is similar for both genders, the incidence pattern is strikingly different. At the time women develop coronary heart disease they are approxi-

Table 1.1. Annual mortality rate by age and gender in the United States (per 100,000 population; WHO Statistics 1997)

	Cardiovascular disease	Myocardial infarction	Ischemic heart disease
Men 65–74 years	104,931 (1269)	28,729 (347)	30,154 (364)
Women 65–74 years	71,443 (698)	17,236 (168)	17,183 (168)
Men >75 years	242,693 (4227)	52,355 (912)	74,376 (1295)
Women >75 years	381,510 (3878)	69,407 (705)	106,049 (1078)

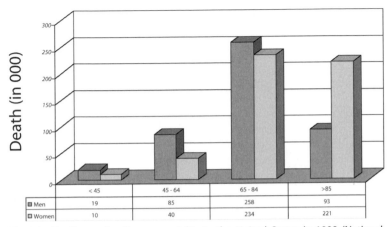

Fig. 1.2. Cardiovascular disease mortality in the United States in 1998 (National Center for Health Statistics and the American Heart Association)

mately 10 years older and at the time of a myocardial infarction they are approximately 20 years older than their male counterparts; thus, CHD in women is definitely a disease of the elderly woman. As already pointed out, before age 75 years, proportionately significantly more men than women die from CVD (Fig. 1.2). This difference is particularly noticeable at younger ages. For example, the male:female ratio is 5.3:1 in individuals 35–44 years and decreases to 1.5:1 in individuals 55–64 years. In other words, 1 of 9 women age 45–65 years develop CHD, but 1 of 3 women age 65 years and older develop it. Taking into account that an increasing number of women live up to 40 years after menopause (the time point at which the risk of coronary artery disease increases at a higher rate), and that in the year 2025 approximately 390 million women will be older than 65 years, the importance of CHD, not only as a public health factor but also with respect to the financial burden for our society, becomes evident.

The CHD is not only responsible for death in women but also for a large percentage of hospitalizations and physical disabilities. Cardiovascular disease is *the* number one diagnosis for women at discharge from the hospital. Thirty-six percent of women 55–64 years, and 55 % of women 75 years and older, have significant limitations in their physical mobility due to CHD.

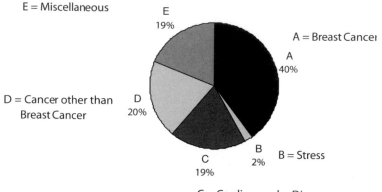

Fig. 1.3. Perceived mortality risk in women (Gallup Poll 1995)

Perception

There is an impressive discrepancy between the actual statistical data and societal perception. A survey taken in 1995 found that 4 of 5 women and one of three general practitioners did not know that CVD is the leading cause of death in women. Most women as well as a large number of physicians still believe that breast cancer is the greatest health threat women face (Fig. 1.3).

Mortality in Myocardial Infarction: Comparison Between Women and Men

In women 40 % of all myocardial infarctions are fatal, and 67 % of all sudden cardiac deaths occur without previous history of CHD. The WHO statistics from 1997 for the United States show that 17,000 women, and 29,000 men age 65–74 years, died from myocardial infarction. But after age 75 years, the data show fatal outcomes for 69,000 women and only 52,000 men (see also Table 1.1). Nevertheless, the number of relatively young women (<65 years) who died from a myocardial infarction is not insignificant (10,200), and 27 % of them were under age 55 years. In women under age 60 years, only 1 in 17 has had a myocardial infarction, whereas the statistic is 1 in 5 for men; however, approximately 20,000 women under 65 years die annually from myocardial infarction. Here also, 30 % of women are younger than 55 years. As demonstrated by the mortality statistics for all cardiovascular diseases, on one hand, the absolute number for women who die from myocardial infarction is high, and on the other hand, the relative number is still lower than for men.

The probability of dying from a myocardial infarction is much higher for women than for men. Closer inspection of the data reveals, however, that at the point of the infarction women are older and suffer from more concomitant illnesses such as hypertension, diabetes mellitus, and hyperlipidemia. After statistical inclusion of these variables, it becomes evident that age and risk factors are primarily, though not exclusively, responsible for the higher mortality rate.

International Comparisons

Since the end of the 1960s a slow but continuous decrease in cardiovascular mortality has been observed for men as well as for women in most European countries and for men in the United States; however, in the United States this trend does not exist for women. On the contrary, cardiovascular mortality has increased (Fig. 1.4). In most European countries, however, cardiovascular mortality is decreasing by 1.5 % per year and the decrease is more pronounced in women than in men. Exceptions are the Central European countries such as Russia, Hungary, Czech Republic (formerly Czechoslovakia), former Yugoslavia, Poland, and former East Germany, where actually an increase in cardiovascular mortality has been shown (Fig. 1.5).

Interestingly, there are great variations among the individual countries, but the correlation between men and women remains the same independent of the country; thus, in countries with a high rate of CHD in the male population a comparably high rate is seen in women, and vice versa; thus, the probability of a woman from an eastern European country dying from CHD is six times higher than that of a man from Japan. It is obvious that environmental factors play a decisive role, more so than genetic disposition and geographic location. This rationale is supported by the fact that even countries that are in close geographical proximity (e.g., Germany and Belgium) clearly show differences in mortality rates. Another proof of the "environmental theory" is found in the trends evident over

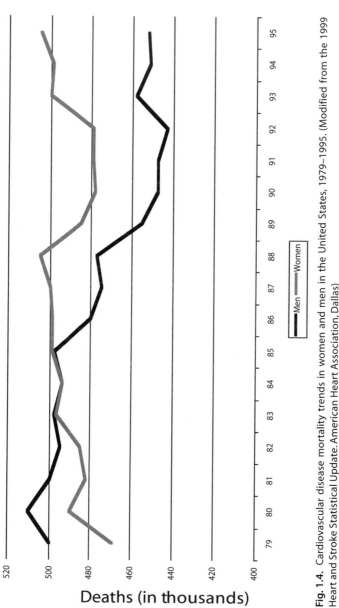

Fig. 1.4. Cardiovascular disease mortality trends in women and men in the United States, 1979–1995. (Modified from the 1999 Heart and Stroke Statistical Update. American Heart Association, Dallas)

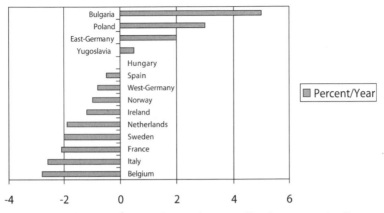

Fig. 1.5. Annual change in cardiovascular mortality in women in Europe, 1970–1992. (Modified from Sans et al. 1997)

time: both in the United States and in England – the countries with the highest rates of CHD from 1950–1954 – the incidence of CHD has been decreasing steadily over the past 20 years, whereas it has been increasing dramatically in eastern European countries. Furthermore, studies in immigrant populations support the "environmental theory": the incidence of CHD in Japanese women living in the United States is twice as high as that of Japanese women living in Japan.

In addition, it has been demonstrated that age-specific mortality is dependent on socioeconomic status, with the highest mortality rates being found in the lowest socioeconomic sectors.

Thus, whichever factors are the actual cause for the differences in mortality in the various countries, their influence is largely independent of gender; instead, these factors affect women and men equally in terms of number, age, and degree.

◆ Summary

Cardiovascular disease remains the leading cause of death in women in the Western world. Approximately 50 % of all deaths are caused by CHD including myocardial infarction and stroke; however, numerous studies over the past 30 years primarily conducted in middle-aged men have led to the misconception that CHD is a disease of men. While it is true that the overall death rate caused by coronary artery disease is similar for both genders, the incidence pattern is strikingly different. At the time women develop CHD they are approximately 10 years older and at the time of a myocardial infarction they are approximately 20 years older than their male counterparts. Despite a worldwide decrease in cardiovascular mortality, this trend is not evident in numerous countries and – most alarmingly – cardiovascular mortality in women in the United States is on the rise.

The "MONItoring CArdiovascular Disease" Project of the WHO (WHO MONICA Project)

The reason(s) for the worldwide decline in deaths from cardiovascular causes are unclear. Possible explanations are a reduction in the incidence of cardiovascular disease and/or in the deaths per individual case. This reversal of the trend might be due to changes in the cardiovascular risk profile of the population (e.g., changes in smoking habits) as well as a simultaneous improvement in therapies (e.g., new blood pressure medications, use of thrombolytic therapy in acute myocardial infarction). To help clarify which of these factors (changes in risk profile and/or improved therapy) might have led to the decrease in cardiovascular lethality, the WHO initiated the MONICA Project in the mid-1980s.

The WHO MONICA Project is the largest and most extensive study ever carried out to investigate the epidemiology of CHD. The main goals of the study were to investigate why the incidence of CHD is increasing in some countries while decreasing in others, and secondly, whether these variations are due primarily to changes in the four classic risk factors (cigarette smoking, high blood pressure, high cholesterol levels, and obesity) or could be attributed to improvements in treatment. A total of 7 million men and women 35–64 years in age from 21 countries (primarily from Europe, also three countries from Asia and two from North America) were included in the study. Study subjects from the individual countries were further divided into subgroups (populations) according to geographical and ethnic criteria. The duration of the study was 10 years (mid-1980s to mid-1990s). Among the factors which were assessed as to their influence on the incidence and mortality rate of CHD were the presence of one or more of the four classic risk factors, the frequency of coronary bypass operations and need for thrombolytic therapy, and use of aspirin, beta-blockers, and angiotensin-converting enzyme inhibitors.

The following data relevant to gender-specific differences were acquired:

1. There was a decrease in the incidence of CHD on average; however, this trend was more pronounced in men, contrary to reports by the Task Force of the European Society of Cardiology on Cardiovascular Mortality and Morbidity Statistics for the study period 1970–1992.

2. A decrease in the risk factors smoking, hypertension, and hyperlipidemia was observed in almost all populations (except for some eastern European countries). Body mass index was increased, however, in most of the populations, in particular for men. There was a wider variation spread for women. The decrease in risk factors was more pronounced in men than in women; in particular, more men than women had stopped smoking.

The decrease in cardiovascular mortality was unrelated to gender and due primarily to a decrease in the incidence of CHD rather than a decrease in mortality (Tunstall-Pedoe et al. 2000). Unexpectedly, for both sexes there was only a weak correlation between the decrease in risk factors and incidence and mortality of CHD (Kuulasmaa et al. 2000). Nevertheless, the correlation was more pronounced in women than in men. The general decrease in cardiovascular mortality was only *partly* attributable to a modification of risk factors. On the other hand, a strong correlation could be observed between use of new therapeutic measures and/or secondary preventive measures and the decrease in cardiac events.

Many questions still remain unanswered. Primary and secondary prevention, and especially improved drug therapy, play an essential role in the decrease in cardiovascular mortality, but these factors cannot explain the general reduction of CHD observed in the industrialized world (with few exceptions and significant differences between eastern and western countries).

References

American Heart Association (2001) Heart and stroke statistical update. American Heart Association 2000, Dallas/TX, American Heart Association Web site. Statistics. http://www.amcericanheart.org

Brett KM, Madans JH (1995) Long-term survival after coronary heart disease: comparisons between men and women in a national sample. Ann Epidemiol 5:25–32

Centers for Disease Control (1992) Coronary heart disease incidence, by sex-United States, 1971–1987. MMWR Morb Mortal Wkly Rep 41(SS-2):526

Khaw KT (1999) Epidemiology of Coronary Heart Disease in Women. In: Julian DG, Wenger NK (eds) Women and Heart Disease. Dunitz, London, pp 7–20

Kuulasmaa K, Tunstall-Pedoe H, Dobson A et al. (2000) Estimation of contribution of changes in classic risk factors to trends in coronary-event rates across the WHO MONICA Project populations. Lancet 355:675–687

Mosca L, Manson JE, Sutherland SE, Langer RD, Manolio T, Barrett-Connor E (1997) Cardiovascular Disease in Women. A Statement for Healthcare Professionals From the American Heart Association. Circulation 96:2468–2482

National Center for Health Statistics (1991) Health: United States – 1990. U.S. Public Health Services, Centers for Disease Control, Hyattsville/MD

Pensky JL, JetteAM, Branch LG et al. (1990) The Framingham Disability Study: relationship of various coronary heart disease manifestations to disability in older persons living in the community. Am J Public Health 80:1363

Sans S, Kesteloot H, Kromhout D on behalf of the Task Force (1997) The burden of cardiovascular diseases mortality in Europe. Task Force of the European Society of Cardiology on Cardiovascular Mortality and Morbidity Statistics in Europe. Eur Heart J 18:1231–1248

Statistisches Bundesamt 1999, Web site http://www.statistik-bund.de

Tunstall-Pedoe H, Vanuzzo D, Hobbs M et al. (2000) Estimation of contribution of changes in coronary care to improving survival, event rates, and coronary heart disease mortality across the WHO MONICA Project populations. Lancet 355:688–700

Wenger NK (1997) Coronary heart disease in women: evolving knowledge is dramatically changing clinical care. In: Julian DG, Wenger NK (eds) Women and Heart Disease. Dunitz, London, p 21

WHO-Statistics. http://www-nt.who.int/whosis/statistics/

WHO Statistik 1997, Web site http://www.who.de

Cardiovascular Risk Factors and the Development of Coronary Heart Disease in Women

Smoking 16

Dyslipidemia 17

Lipoprotein (a) 19

Diabetes Mellitus 20

Insulin Resistance and Polycystic Ovary Syndrome . . . 21

Family History of Coronary Heart Disease
or Genetic Disposition 23

Hypertension 23

Sedentary Lifestyle 24

Obesity 25

Homocysteine 26

High sensitivity C-reactive Protein 27

Risk Factors Unique to Women 28

References 30

The following risk factors are associated with a high prevalence of coronary heart disease, both in men and women:

- Age
- Family history of coronary heart disease
- Smoking
- Hypertension
- Dyslipidemia
- Diabetes mellitus

However, risk factors may have a different relative importance in men and women. For example, diabetes mellitus and smoking carry a greater incremental risk in women than in men. A risk factor unique to women is menopause. Natural menopause or any other cause of estrogen deprivation (i.e., ovariectomy) has been shown to have a substantial increase in risk for coronary heart disease.

Only 30 % of all women in the United States do not have any cardiovascular risk factors at all. Thirty percent of women age 20–74 years are found to have hypertension, 25 % hyperlipidemia, 25 % obesity, and another 25 % of women smoke. The prevalence of all risk factors, in particular obesity, smoking, and lack of exercise, is especially high in women with less favorable socioeconomic and educational status. With increasing age there is a crossover of risk characteristics between men and women such that hypertension and dyslipidemia are more prevalent in young men than young women but become more prevalent in elderly women than in elderly men. In contrast to the dramatic decrease in cardiovascular risk factors over the past 20 years in men, there has been little change for women, most likely due to the fact that physicians focus more on risk factors in men and therefore men receive a higher level of preventive care.

❶ Perhaps the most important risk factor for coronary artery disease is the misperception that coronary artery disease is a men's disease.

Despite the fact that this misconception is gradually being corrected by both physicians and patients, it still has important impact on all aspects of prevention, diagnosis, and therapy. As long as a woman does not consider coronary heart disease as a threat to her health, she will not change her lifestyle for risk modification and will not seek medical attention for symptoms. In order to reduce cardiovascular morbidity and mortality in women, the importance of coronary artery disease in the female population has to be recognized.

The American Heart Association (AHA) highlights the importance of a gender-specific approach to coronary artery disease since it developed algorithms for a gender-specific risk assessment (Grundy et al. 1999; Mosca et al. 1999). Furthermore, the American Heart Association and the American College of Cardiology developed guidelines for primary and secondary prevention of coronary artery disease in women, thus recognizing gender differences in coronary prevention as well (Fig. 2.1).

Despite the fact that classic risk factors play an important role in the development of coronary heart disease, there is no strong correlation between cardiovascular risk and the incidence of cardiovascular events. The reasons have not yet been clarified; however "newer" risk factors such as (a) markers of fibrinolytic function (e.g., tissue type plasminogen activator (t-PA) and plasminogen activator inhibitor 1 (PAI-1), and factor 7 and 8, (b) vitamins (e.g., vitamin B and D), (c) markers of inflammation (leukocytes, C-reactive protein, adhesion molecules), and (d) infection (*Chlamydia pneumonia, Helicobacter pylori*, herpes virus, cytomegalovirus) may play an important role.

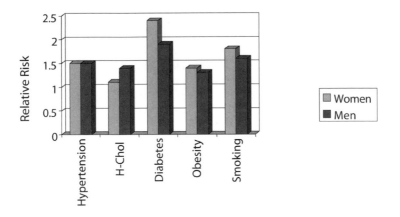

H-Chol = Hypercholesterolemia

Fig. 2.1. Coronary heart disease incidence by gender and risk factors. (Modified from Centers for Disease Control 1992)

Smoking

Smoking is the most preventable cause of death. It accounts for approximately 50 % of all avoidable deaths and for 25 % of cardiovascular diseases. In comparison with men, women who smoke have a threefold increased risk of fatal coronary artery disease and nonfatal myocardial infarction. In addition, women who smoke will experience a myocardial infarction at an earlier age than men.

There is a clear dose–response relationship between the number of cigarettes currently smoked and risk of coronary heart disease. The risk is particularly high in women who started smoking before age 15 years. The Nurse's Health Study found that the relative risk (RR) of coronary heart disease was 2.1 for smokers of 1–14 cigarettes per day and 6.0 for those smoking 25 or more cigarettes per day. This risk is present even with passive smoking, minimal exposure (5 cigarettes per day), smoking of low-yield cigarettes, and chewing of tobacco. Epidemiological data indicate that there is a synergistic effect of smoking and the use of oral contraceptive pills, especially in women over age 35 years. Although smoking rates in the United States are falling overall, they have declined more slowly in women than in men (50 vs 33 %). In eastern Europe and in some developing countries, smoking rates in women are even on the rise, leading to increased cardiovascular mortality. Furthermore, the prevalence of daily smoking among female high school seniors in the United States is increasing (Fried and Becker 1993). Given the fact that most of the young women take birth control pills as well, it is of uttermost importance to educate the public and to support smoking cessation programs. Smoking leads to an earlier menopause (on average 1.5–2 years earlier), increasing further the risk of coronary heart disease (Shapiro et al. 1979).

Coronary heart disease decreases rapidly after cessation of smoking, independent of age, number of cigarettes smoked, and years of smoking. Smoking cessation benefits even women with documented coronary heart disease. After 3–5 years, the risk level falls to levels consistent with those who have never smoked.

❶ **Women experience more difficulty in quitting smoking. A possible explanation is the fact that women more often smoke to lose or maintain body weight (Hermanson et al. 1988).**

Dyslipidemia

Lipoproteins play an important role in the development and rupture of atherosclerotic plaques.

The most important serum lipids are:
- Cholesterol
- Triglycerides
- Fatty acids
- Phospholipids

Lipids are water insoluble. In order to disperse in the aqueous blood system, lipids are generally transported as part of particles, termed lipoproteins; these are composed of protein, phospholipids, triglycerides, and cholesterol. Various proteins located on the surface (apoproteins) allow interaction with other biological systems.

Lipoproteins are either classified with respect to their density, to their electrophoretic mobility (Fredrickson classification), or with respect to their apoproteins. The most commonly used system is based on density. Particles which are dense and relatively cholesterol rich are called low-density lipoproteins (LDL). High-density lipoprotein (HDL) is relatively cholesterol poor. Triglyceride-rich particles are termed very low-density lipoproteins (VLDL). Large transport particles, derived from an intestinal source, are termed chylomicrons.

Cholesterol levels are determined by the amount of hepatic LDL receptors. For example, a meal rich in cholesterol downregulates the production of LDL receptors and leads to hypercholesterolemia.

By definition, hypercholesterolemia is present when serum cholesterol levels are greater than 200 mg/dl, independent of gender. Since Framingham, it is well known that elevated cholesterol levels are associated with a higher risk of cardiovascular disease. The relative risk (RR) for men age 30–49 years with cholesterol levels of 240–259 mg/dl in comparison with men with normal cholesterol levels is 1.71. A cholesterol over 260 mg/dl is associated with an RR of 2.2. Elevated total cholesterol and LDL levels are a less important risk factor in women than in men, in particular in women under the age of 65 years (Table 2.1); however, HDL plays a major role in risk assessment of coronary heart disease in women. The HDL is inversely related to the risk of coronary heart disease and is a significant predictor of a decreased risk (Denke 1999; Miller 1994).

Table 2.1. Relation between dyslipidemia and risk of coronary heart disease. (Modified from Walsh 1999)

Relative risk[a]	Total cholesterol[b]	LDL[c]	HDL[d]
Women			
<65 years	2.44	3.27	2.13
>65 years	1.12	1.13	1.75
Men			
<65 years	1.73	1.92	2.31
>65 years	1.32	1.51	1.09

[a] Data derived from 86,000 women
[b] Comparison of total cholesterol >240 mg/dl with total cholesterol <200 mg/dl
[c] Comparison of LDL-C >160 mg/dl with LDL-C <140 mg/dl
[d] Comparison of HDL-C <50 mg/dl with HDL-C >60 mg/dl

Epidemiological studies could not define a lower limit of cholesterol level that prohibits the development of coronary heart disease; however, most secondary prevention studies have convincingly shown that cholesterol reduction is associated with improved clinical outcome. For example, in men a 1 % reduction in the serum cholesterol level yields a two to three times reduction in the risk of coronary disease. Several epidemiological studies found a similar relationship in women. Unfortunately, data from randomized trials are not yet available.

The HDL plays a major role in cholesterol clearance. Furthermore, it improves endothelial function and has antioxidant properties. Independent of gender-elevated HDL levels (normal value 35–54 mm/dl) are associated with decreased risk of coronary heart disease. There is a 40–50 % reduction in risk with each 10 mg/dl increase in HDL. The relative importance of HDL levels is higher in women than in men. Low HDL levels are associated with an especially high risk in women. The risk of nonfatal myocardial infarction or cardiovascular mortality increases by 50 % in women with an HDL under 35 mg/dl in comparison with men with the same HDL level. The most common with low HDL level associated dyslipidemia is hypoalphalipoproteinemia, defined as an HDL below tenth percentile which is less than approximately 29 mg/dl for middle-aged men and less than 38 mg/dl for middle-aged women. It almost always leads to premature coronary heart disease.

The HDL levels are higher in women than in men across the lifespan (approximately 10 mg/dl higher). The HDL levels decrease only insignificantly after menopause. During their childbearing years, women have significantly lower levels of low-density lipoprotein (LDL) than men, but after menopause levels of LDL exceed those seen in elderly men. This accounts for the increasing total cholesterol levels observed in postmenopausal women; thus, postmenopausal women have a more atherogenic lipid profile then premenopausal women which may in part explain the increased cardiovascular morbidity and mortality of the elderly woman.

According to the National Cholesterol Education Program (NCEP) the ratio of total to HDL cholesterol has been shown to provide a more accurate measure of coronary risk than total cholesterol alone. A ratio less than 3.5 is associated with low risk, a ratio over 7 with high risk.

Hypertriglyceridemia is defined as serum triglyceride level greater than 200 mg/dl. Hypertriglyceridemia is an independent risk factor for coronary heart disease in women, especially for women over the age of 65 years (Criqui et al. 1993; LaRosa 1997). High triglyceride levels and low HDL levels tend to coincide. Furthermore, hypertriglyceridemia is often associated with diabetes mellitus or genetic dyslipoproteinemias. The complex interactions between triglycerides and other lipid parameters may obscure the impact of triglycerides in the development of coronary heart disease. One example of hypertriglyceridemia with a high risk of coronary heart disease is familiar hypertriglyceridemia (type-IV dyslipidemia of the Fredrickson classification). This type of lipid disorder is frequently associated with impaired glucose tolerance and hyperuricemia.

Lipoprotein (a)

Lipoprotein (a) (Lp/a) is an LDL particle and a protein with structural similarities to those of plasminogen. Elevated Lp/a levels are associated with decreased endothelial-dependent arterial relaxation. Since Lp(a) serum levels increase after menopause, a relationship between estrogen and Lp(a) has been discussed (Shlipak et al. 2000); however, the predictive nature of Lp(a) in the development of coronary heart disease in women is still controversial. In men several observational studies demonstrated that Lp(a) levels greater than 30 mg/dl are associated with a threefold higher risk of coronary heart disease and furthermore with a higher risk of restenosis after balloon angioplasty. The Framingham study has reported that Lp(a) greater than 30 mg/dl is a strong independent predictor of myocardial infarction, intermittent claudication, and cerebral vascular disease (Bostom et al. 1994). Coleman et al. (1992) did not confirm these data, but since the study had inadequate statistical power a true association could have been missed.

Diabetes Mellitus

Diabetes mellitus (regardless of whether insulin dependent or not) essentially eliminates any cardioprotective effect regardless of gender, even for premenopausal women (Grundy et al. 1999; Jousilahti et al. 1999). In other words, the risk of coronary heart disease in premenopausal diabetic women is identical to that of nondiabetic men. Furthermore, diabetes mellitus is a stronger coronary heart disease risk factor in women than in men (Table 2.2). Mortality rates for coronary heart disease are three to seven times higher for diabetic vs nondiabetic women, compared with rates that are two to three times higher for diabetic vs nondiabetic men. Based on these data, the American Heart Association came to the conclusion that diabetes mellitus in women has twice the weight than that in men when calculating coronary artery disease risk (Grundy et al 1999).

The Nurses' Health Study demonstrated that the incidence of diabetes was less among women who exercised regularly; therefore, a regular exercise regimen should be recommended as a preventative strategy, particularly for women at high risk for diabetes (i.e., women who have had gestational diabetes or women with a genetic disposition).

Non-insulin-dependent diabetes mellitus is frequently associated with obesity (particularly central obesity), hypertension, and insulin resistance. This cluster of risk factors may be related to high circulating insulin levels.

Diabetes mellitus not only imparts a higher risk but also a less favorable outcome of clinical coronary events. In the Framingham cohort, the risk of death and nonfatal myocardial infarction for a diabetic vs a nondiabetic woman was 4.4 fold increased compared with a 2.4 fold increase for

Table 2.2. Gender-based relative risk of coronary heart disease in patients with insulin-dependent diabetes mellitus. *RR* relative risk

Study	Age (years)	RR in women	RR in men
Framingham[a]	45–74	3.3	1.7
Evans County[b]	>22	2.8	1.0
Rancho Bernardo[c]	40–79	3.5	2.4
Rochester[d]	>30	3.2	2.7
Strong Heart[e]	45–74	4.6	1.8

[a]Kannel and McGee (1979)
[b]Heyden et al. (1980)
[c]Barrett-Connor and Wingard (1983)
[d]Elvebach et al. (1986)
[e]Howard et al. (1995)

a diabetic vs a nondiabetic man. Diabetic women with a myocardial infarction have twice the risk of reinfarction and a fourfold increase in the risk of development of heart failure (Jousilahti et al. 1999). More women then men undergoing coronary artery bypass graft surgery or percutaneous transluminal coronary angioplasty are diabetic which has a substantial impact on less favorable outcome in women.

Insulin Resistance and Polycystic Ovary Syndrome

Under normal conditions intake of carbohydrates stimulates insulin production in the pancreas, which subsequently leads to glucose utilization by muscle and fat cells. In patients with insulin resistance, higher circulating insulin levels for glucose uptake are necessary. Glucose intolerance is present if circulating glucose levels remain high despite increased insulin production. In case hyperinsulinemia is unable to control blood glucose levels, type-II diabetes mellitus is present.

Hyperinsulinemia is an independent risk factor in men and women, independent of impaired glucose tolerance or diabetes mellitus.

Insulin resistance and hyperinsulinemia are frequently associated with numerous abnormalities that are atherogenic (Laws et al. 1993):

- Impaired glucose tolerance
- Diabetes mellitus
- Hypertriglyceridemia
- Hyperuricemia
- Hypertension
- Low HDL
- High LDL

This clustering of risk factors has been termed insulin resistance syndrome (see table).

Characteristics of insulin resistance syndrome

– Insulin resistance	– Small dense LDL
– Hyperinsulinemia	– Hyperuricemia
– Hypertriglyceridemia	– Hypertension
– Low HDL	– Abnormal fibrinolytic activity
– High VLDL	

Weight loss and/or regular physical activity (especially aerobic fitness) have a major positive impact on insulin sensitivity. Regular physical activity lowers the incidence of type-II diabetes mellitus.

Given the fact that central obesity and a sedentary lifestyle is more prevalent in women, insulin resistance and hyperinsulinemia are also more common in women than in men, suggesting a higher risk for women; however, too few studies have examined the relationship of baseline hyperinsulinemia to the incidents of coronary artery disease in women to draw any reliable conclusion.

A condition specific to women that is characterized by insulin resistance and hyperinsulinemia is polycystic ovary syndrome (PCO). Women with PCO not only have hyperinsulinemia, but also elevated levels of circulating androgens and in many cases elevated triglycerides and decreased HDL levels as well (Dunaif et al. 1989; Robinson et al. 1996; Talbott et al. 1995). Cross-sectional studies in women with PCO and angiographic documented coronary heart disease demonstrated that women with PCO had more extensive coronary artery disease than women with normal ovaries (Birdsall et al. 1997); however, no prospective studies are available yet to confirm these data.

Family History of Coronary Heart Disease or Genetic Disposition

A genetic disposition of coronary heart disease is present if parents, siblings, or children have documented coronary heart disease before age 55 years in men, and before age 65 years in women. The Second Joint Task Force of European and Other Societies on Coronary Prevention recommends early screening for risk factors and, if present, preventative measures as soon as possible.

Hypertension

The World Health Organization defines hypertension as blood pressure of 140/90 or above. Hypertension consistently correlates with a higher risk of cardiovascular events (Fig. 2.2). The risk imposed by hypertension increases even further in the presence of other cardiovascular risk factors such as hyperlipidemia, smoking, diabetes mellitus, and obesity (Bittner et al 1993; Hayes and Tayler 1998). According to data from the National Health and Nutrition Examination Survey the prevalence of hypertension in the United States between 1991 and 1994 was 75 % in women and 62 % in men age 18–74 years. Under age 45 years, hypertension is more common in men than in women; however, after age 60 years, the age-associated rise in blood pressure is more pronounced in women than in men (Bittner and Oparil 1993). Seventy percent of women 65 years or older and 80 % of women 75 years or older are hypertensive. After age 80 years the prevalence of hypertension is 14 % higher in women than in men. Furthermore, isolated systolic hypertension is more prevalent among women than among men. Obesity, frequently associated with hypertension, is also strongly linked to the development of hypertension, especially in women.

Left ventricular hypertrophy (LVH) as a sequelae of hypertension is associated with increased cardiovascular morbidity and mortality, independent of gender; however, women with LVH have a greater increase in relative risk than men. The annual incidence of LVH in women with mild hypertension is twice that of women with normal blood pressure. Moderate hypertension increases the incidence tenfold (4–15 fold in men). The

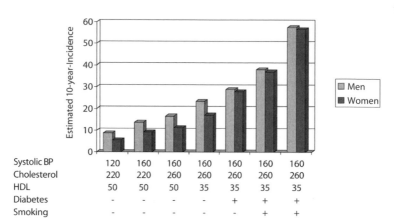

Systolic BP	120	160	160	160	160	160	160
Cholesterol	220	220	260	260	260	260	260
HDL	50	50	50	35	35	35	35
Diabetes	-	-	-	-	+	+	+
Smoking	-	-	-	-	-	+	+

Fig. 2.2. Estimated 10-year risk of coronary heart disease due to hypertension and other cardiovascular risk factors in men and women. (Modified from Anderson et al. 1991)

importance of prevention and control of high blood pressure for prevention of LVH is of the utmost importance.

Sedentary Lifestyle

Sedentary lifestyle is an independent risk factor for coronary heart disease in women. A sedentary lifestyle is most prevalent in women of lower socioeconomic class and education. Physical activity has a positive impact on multiple risk factors. Long-term exercise training results in increased HDL levels, lower triglyceride levels, and less insulin resistance (Kannel and Wilson 1995).

A total of 43 epidemiological studies demonstrated that even leisure time activity (gardening, bicycling, etc.) lowers the risk of coronary heart disease. Despite the fact that 36 of the 43 studies were conducted in men only, a subgroup analysis for women of the remaining 7 studies suggests a 50 % reduction in risk in women (Berlin and Colditz 1990); however, given the small numbers of women included in these studies and the difficulties of measuring physical activity, this data can be an estimate only. Independent of these epidemiological studies, randomized trials could demonstrate that brisk walking 30–45 min three times per week is associated with a significantly reduced risk for cardiovascular events. This is even true for postmenopausal women and women 65 years and older (Lemaitre et al. 1995; Manson et al. 1991). Intense physical activity in elderly women, however, is associated with an increased incidence of muscle and bone injuries. In this patient population moderate activities are the preferred form of exercise.

Obesity

Obesity is defined as a body mass index (BMI) above 25. A BMI above 30 is consistent with marked obesity. Body mass index can be calculated by dividing weight (in kilograms) by height (in meters) squared. For example a woman 165 cm tall who weighs more than 75 kg is significantly obese (BMI of 27.6). Since BMI better defines total body fat mass than weight alone, it has become the preferred way of defining obesity.

The prevalence of obesity has been steadily rising. Thirty-three percent of white women and 50 % of African-American women in the United States are overweight. The prevalence of overweight is clustered in women with less favorable social economic and educational status. In Europe, 25 % of women with documented coronary disease are found to have a BMI over 30 (Second Joint Task Force of European on Coronary Prevention 1998).

The relative risk of myocardial infarction is reduced by 35–60 % in women with normal BMI (<25; Fig 2.3). In contrast, abdominal or central obesity (determined by a waist/hip ratio >0.8) is even a stronger risk factor for coronary artery disease in women than BMI alone. This kind of obesity is often associated with "syndrome x" (or metabolic syndrome) which has been defined as a combination of insulin resistance, hyperglycemia, low HDL, hypertension, and hypertriglyceridemia (Kaplan 1989). These patients frequently have a very small and dense LDL and an unusually high risk of early atherosclerosis (Austin and Shelby 1995).

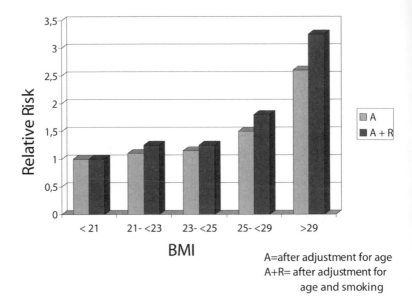

A=after adjustment for age
A+R= after adjustment for
age and smoking

Fig. 2.3. Relation between body mass index (BMI) and the relative risk of coronary heart disease. (From the Nurses' Health Study 1990)

Homocysteine

Homocysteine is a sulfhydryl-containing amino acid derived from the demethylation of dietary methionine. Homocysteine plasma concentrations are determined by diet, age, smoking habits and gender. In general men, smokers and elderly individuals have a higher homocysteine level than women, nonsmokers or young individuals. High plasma homocysteine concentrations (normal values 5–15 μmol/l) are associated with an increased risk of coronary heart disease in men (Stampfer et al. 1998). Gender-specific data are not yet available. There is an inverse relationship between homocysteine levels and plasma levels of folate, vitamin B6, and vitamin B_{12}. Since the Nurses' Health Study demonstrated a significant reduction in cardiovascular disease morbidity and mortality in women with dietary intake of folate and vitamin B_6 (Rimm et al. 1998), elevated homocysteine levels may play a critical role for women as well. Supplementation with these vitamins, in particular folic acid, normalizes plasma homocysteine levels after 4–6 weeks.

High sensitivity C-reactive Protein

Inflammation plays an important role in all phases of atherosclerosis; therefore, it is not surprising that several markers of systemic inflammation have also proven useful for cardiovascular risk prediction. Among the inflammatory markers and lipid markers of risk, high sensitivity C-reactive protein (hs-CRP) has been proven to be the single best predictor of future vascular events in women (including myocardial infarction, stroke, sudden cardiac death). In the Women's Health Study even mildly elevated plasma levels of hs-CRP were associated with increased cardiovascular risk. Women with the highest quartile of hs-CRP had a fivefold to sevenfold increased risk of cardiac and vascular events over a 3-year follow-up in comparison with women with hs-CRP values in the lowest quartile (Ridker et al. 2000). Moreover, this difference in risk was most striking in women with documented myocardial infarction or stroke. On the other

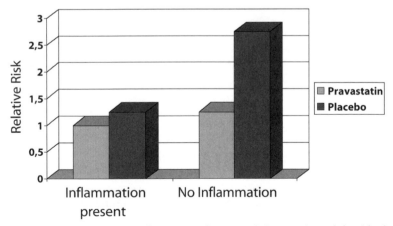

Fig. 2.4. Relation between inflammation, therapy with Pravastatin, and the risk of coronary events after myocardial infarction. (Modified from Ridker et al. 1998)

hand, even in women with low risk elevated plasma levels of hs-CRP appear to add to the predictive value of plasma lipid measurements (Ridker et al. 1998). Moreover, in multivariate analysis, only studies which included hs-CRP for risk stratification were more powerful than studies which relied on lipid profile and total cholesterol/HDL-C ratio only.

In the Cholesterol And Recurrent Event Trial (CARE) long-term treatment with pravastatin (a hydroxy-methyl-glutaryl-CoA-reductase inhibitor) of patients with elevated hs-CRP levels was associated with a significant reduction in cardiovascular events (Fig. 2.4). In this trial elevated hs-CRP levels were more closely correlated with cardiovascular events than total cholesterol levels. There was a 54 % risk reduction in patients with abnormal hs-CRP in contrast to 25 % of patients with normal hs-CRP. Despite the fact that there was no subgroup analysis for women with respect to hs-CRP levels and statin therapy, there was an overall greater risk reduction in women than in men. These findings suggest that lipid lowering with statin drugs attenuates the inflammatory processes that undermine stability, and hence reduces cardiovascular risk.

Risk Factors Unique to Women

Menopause

Natural menopause or any kind of estrogen deficiency (i.e., secondary to ovariectomy or chemotherapy) is associated with a higher risk of coronary artery disease. Estrogen deficiency not only has a negative impact on several cardiovascular risk factors (i.e., increase in total cholesterol, LDL cholesterol, Lp(a), homocysteine, PAI-1, decrease in HDL) but also decreases aortic root elasticity. Data from the Nurses' Health Study showed that in women with bilateral oophorectomy the coronary risk was 1.5 times that in premenopausal women of comparable age (Fig. 2.5). Taking into account that women now survive well beyond their reproductive years and spend approximately one-third of their life in the post-menopausal state, menopause and the risk of coronary heart disease in women has become an increasing rather than a waning problem.

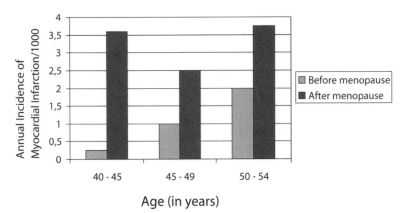

Fig. 2.5. Menopause and the risk of coronary heart disease. (Modified data from Kannel and Wilson 1995)

Oral Contraception

Epidemiological studies on combined (estrogen and progestin) oral contraceptives with high (50–150 μg/d) or medium (35–50 μg/d) estrogen doses uniformly showed an increase in risk of myocardial infarction, particularly in cigarette smoking women. Exogenous estrogen is associated with increased rates of intravascular thrombosis, including deep vein thrombosis, pulmonary embolism, as well as myocardial infarction and stroke. The risk of the newer low-dose preparations (20–35 μg/d) still remains unclear in nonsmoking women. Most likely they are not associated with an increased risk of myocardial infarction or stroke. However, the incidence of pathological thrombosis remains high among smoking women over the age of 35 years; therefore, in these women, smoking cessation or alternative methods of contraception are recommended (Fig. 2.6). In addition, oral contraception has a negative impact on high blood pressure; however, after discontinuation of the drug, normalization of blood pressure is the rule.

 Summary

The prevalence of coronary heart disease is associated with the classic risk factors, both in men and women; however, risk factors may have a different

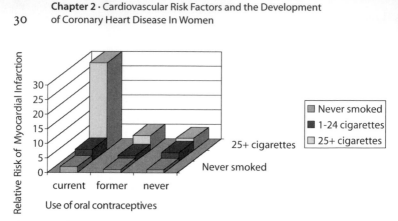

Fig. 2.6. Relation between smoking, use of oral contraceptives, and the risk of myocardial infarction. (Modified from Rosenberg et al. 1985)

relative importance in men and women. Diabetes mellitus and smoking carry a greater incremental risk in women than in men, in particular in women who use oral contraceptives. Natural menopause or any kind of estrogen deficiency (i.e., secondary to ovariectomy or chemotherapy) is the strongest gender-specific risk factor for coronary artery disease. A particularly female syndrome associated with substantial risk is the PCO. The single best marker for future vascular events in women is the hs-CRP. Evaluation of risk requires a gender-specific approach.

References

Anderson KM, Wilson PW, Odell PM, Kannel WB (1991) An updated coronary risk profile. Circulation 83:357–363]

Austin MA, Shelby JV (1995) LDL subclass phenotypes and the risk factors of the insulin resistance syndrome. Int J Obes 19(Suppl 1):S22–26

Barrett-Connor E, Wingard DL (1983) Sex differential in ischemic heart disease mortality in diabetics: a prospective population-based study. Am J Epidemiol 118:489–496

Berlin JA, Colditz GA (1990) A meta-analysis of physical activity in the prevention of coronary heart disease. Am J Epidemiol 132:612–628

Bittner V, Oparil S (1993) Hypertension. In: Douglas PS (ed) Cardiovascular health and disease in women. Saunders, Philadelphia, p 63

Birdsall MA, Farquhar CM, White HD (1997) Association between polycystic ovaries and extent of coronary artery disease in women having cardiac catheterization. Ann Intern Med 126:32–35

Bostom AG, Gagnon DR, Cupples A et al. (1994) A prospective investigation of elevated lipoprotein a detectedby electrophoresis and cardiovascular disease in women: The Framingham heart study. Circulation 90:1688

Castelli WP, Garrison RJ, Wilson PWF et al. (1986) Incidence of coronary heart disease and lipoprotein cholesterol levels: The Framingham study. JAMA 256:2835–2838

Centers of Disease Control (1992) Coronary heart disease incidence by sex – United States. MMWR Morb Mortal Wkly Rep 41(SS-2):526]

Coleman MP, Key TJA, Wang EY et al. (1992) A prospective study of obesity, lipids, apolipoproteins and ischaemic heart disease in women. Artherosclerosis 92:177–185

Criqui MH, Heiss G, Cohn R et al. (1993) Plasma triglycerides level and mortality from coronary heart disease. N Engl J Med 328:1220–1225

Denke MA (1999) Primary prevention of coronary heart disease in postmenopausal women. Am J Med 107 (2 A).48 S

Dunaif A, Segal KR, Futterweit W, Dobrjansky A (1989) Profound peripheral insulin resistance, independent of obesity, in polycystic ovary syndrome. Diabetes 28:1165–1174

Eaker ED, Castelli WP (1987) Coronary heart disease and it's risk factors among women in the Framingham Study. In: Eaker ED, Paker B, Wenger N et al. (eds) Coronary Heart Disease in Women. Haymarket Doyma, New York, p 122

Elveback LR, Connaolly DC, Melton LJ III (1986) Coronary heart disease in residents of Rochester, Minnesota. VII. Incidence, 1950 through 1982. Mayo Clin Proc 61:896–900

Fried LP, Becker DM (1993) Smoking and cardiovascular disease. In: Douglas PS (ed) Cardiovascular Health and Disease in Women. Saunders, Philadelphia, p 217

Grundy SM, Pasternak R, Greenland P et al. (1999) Assessment of cardiovascular risk by use of multiple risk-factor assessment equations: A statement for healthcare professionals from the American Heart Association and the American College of Cardiology. Circulation 100:1481

Hayes SN, Taler SJ (1998) Hypertension in women: current understanding of gender differences. Mayo Clin Proc 73:157

Heyden S, Heiss G, Bartel AG et al. (1980) Sex differences in coronary mortality among diabetics in Evans County, Georgia. J Chron Dis 33:265–273

Hermanson B, Omenn GS, Kronmal RA et al. (1988) Beneficial six-year outcome of smoking cessation in older men and women with coronary artery disease: Results from CASS registry. N Engl J Med 319:1365

Howard BV, Lee ET, Cowan LD et al. (1995) Coronary heart disease prevalence and its relation to risk factors in American Indians: The Strong Heart Study. Am J Epidemiol 142:254–268

Howard BV, Cowan LD, Haffner SM (1997) Women, Diabetes, Lipoproteins, and the Risk for Coronary Heart Disease. In: Forte TM (ed) Hormonal, metabolic, and cellular influences on cardiovascular disease in women. Futura Publishing Company, Armonk/NY, S 262]

Jousilahti P, Vartiainen E, Tuomilehto J, Puska P (1999) Sex, age, cardiovascular risk factors, and coronary heart disease: A prospective follow-up study of 14.786 middle-aged men and women in Finland. Circulation 99:1165

Kannel WB, McGee DL (1979) Diabetes and cardiovascular disease: The Framingham study. JAMA 241:2035–2038

Kannel WB, Wilson PWF (1995) Risk factors that attenuate the female coronary disease advantage. Arch Intern Med 155:57

Kaplan NM (1989) The deadly quartet: upper-body obesity, glucose intolerance, hypertryglyceridemia, and hypertension. Arch Intern Med 149:1514

Kushi LH, Fee RM, Folsom AR et al. (1997) Physical activity and mortality in post-menopausal women. JAMA 277:1287

LaRosa JC (1993) Lipoproteins and lipid disorders. In: Douglas PS (ed) Cardiovascular health and disease in women. Saunders, Philadelphia, p 175

LaRosa JC (1997) Triglycerides and coronary risk in women and the elderly. Arch Intern Med 157:961

Laws A, King AC, Haskell WL, Reaven GM (1993) Metabolic and behavioral covariates of high-density lipoprotein cholesterol and triglycerides concentrations in post-menopausal women. J Am Geriatr Soc 41:1289–1294

Lemaitre RN, Heckbert SR, Psaty BM et al. (1995) Leisure-time physical activity and the risk of nonfatal myocardial infarction in postmenopausal women. Arch Intern Med 155:2302

Manson JE, Colditz GA, Stampfer MJ et al. (1991) A prospective study of maturity-onset diabetes mellitus and risk of coronary heart disease and stroke in women. Arch Intern Med 151:1141–1147

Manson JE, Hu FB, Rich-Edwards JW et al. (1999) A prospective study of walking as compared with vigorous exercise in the prevention of coronary heart disease in women. N Engl J Med 341:650

Miller VT (1994) Lipids, lipoproteins women and cardiovascular disease. Artherosclerosis 108:S73

Mosca L, Grundy SM, Judelson D et al. (1999) Guide to preventative cardiology for women. Circulation 99:2480

Mosca L, Manson JE, Sutherland SE et al. (1997) Cardiovascular disease in women: A statement for healthcare professionals from the AHA. Circulation 96:2468

National Cholesterol Education Program (1994) Detection, evaluation, and treatment of high blood cholesterol in adults (Adult Treatment Panel II). Circulation 89:1329–1445

Ridker PM, Buring JE, Shih J et al. (1998) Prospective study of C-reactive protein and the risk of future cardiovascular events among apparently healthy women. Circulation 98:731–733

References

Ridker PM, Rifai N, Pfeffer MA et al. (1999) Long-term effects of Pravastatin on plasma concentration of C-reactive protein. Circulation 100:230–235

Ridker PM, Hennekens CH, Buring JE et al. (2000) C-reactive protein and other markers of inflammation in the prediction of cardiovascular disease in women. N Engl J Med 342:836–843

Rimm EB, Willett WC, Hu FB et al. (1998) Folate and vitamin B6 from diet and supplements in relation to risk of coronary heart disease among women. JAMA 279:359–364

Robinson S, Henderson AD, Gelding SV et al. (1996) Dyslipidaemia is associated with insulin resistance in women with polycystic ovaries. Clin Endocrinol 44:277–284

Rosenberg L, Kaufman DW, Helmrich SP, Miller DR, Stolley PD, Shapiro S (1985) Myocardial infarcation and cigarette smoking in women younger than 50 years of age. JAMA 253(20): 2965–2969]

Second Joint Task Force of European and other societies on Coronary Prevention (1998) Prevention of coronary heart disease in clinical practice. Eur Heart J 19:1434–1503

Shapiro S, Sloane D, Rosenberg L et al. (1979) Oral contraceptive use in relation to myocardial infarction. Lancet 1:743

Shlipak MG, Simon JA, Vittinghoff E et al. (2000) Estrogen and progestin, lipoprtein (a), and the risk of recurrent coronary heart disease events after menopause. JAMA 283:1845–1852

Stampfer MJ, Malinow MR, Willett WC (1998) A prospective study of plasma homocyst(e)ine and risk of myocardial infarction in U. S. physicians. JAMA 279:359–364

Talbott E, Guzick D, Clerici A et al. (1995) Coronary heart disease risk factors in women with polycystic ovary syndrome. Aterioscler Thromb Vasc Biol 15:821–826

Van Poppel G, Kardinaal A, Princen H, Kok FJ (1994) Antioxidants and coronary heart disease. Ann Med 26:429–434

Walsh JME (1999) Lipids. In: Charney P (ed) Coronary artery disease in women: What all physicians need to know. American College of Physician Press, Philadelphia, p 104

Pathophysiology
of Coronary Heart Disease
and the Effects of Estrogen

Basics 36

Effects of Estrogen 38

References 44

Basics

Atherosclerosis of the coronary arteries is the underlying pathophysiological mechanism of coronary heart disease (CHD) and is the same for both genders. There are numerous different theories with regard to the genesis of atherosclerosis. The most commonly held and most credible theory is the "response-to-injury" hypothesis by R. Ross according to which various types of injuries in the endothelium and in vascular smooth muscle cells (SMCs) lead to an exaggerated inflammatory fibroproliferative reaction in the vessel wall with subsequent plaque formation.

Plaque Formation and Significance of Plaques in CHD

Unrelated to the gender, any damage to endothelial function (e.g., due to risk factors such as smoking, diabetes, insulin resistance, etc.) leads to changes in the release of vasoactive substances, to increased uptake of lipoproteins by the intima, and to expression of glycoproteins on the endothelium cell surface which serves as adhesion molecules for monocytes and T-lymphocytes. As a result of the deposit of lipids, the monocytes change into foam cells which subsequently form fatty streaks together with lymphocytes. Intermediate lesions occur after the proliferation of SMCs and microphages, and complex so-called fibrous plaques form after the accumulation of lipids in the cells and connective tissue matrix. They are composed of a nucleus rich in lipids and filled with necrotic substance and a fibrous capsule containing a few SMCs. Initially, the coronary artery expands via plaque formation toward the adventitia. Later the plaques grow in the direction of the lumen, causing vessel stenosis (Fig. 3.1).

Until recently it was assumed that stable as well as unstable angina and myocardial infarction were caused by a severe (i.e., >75 % narrowing of the lumen) arteriosclerotic coronary stenosis; thus, therapy was based primarily on the angiographic identification of the culprit stenosis with the goal of coronary intervention; however, the majority of ST-elevation and non-ST-elevation myocardial infarctions occur in stenoses <50 %. In recent years it has become evident that factors other than the severity of the stenosis play a decisive role in unstable angina and myocardial infarctions. Occlusive coronary thrombosis is neither caused by the size of the plaque nor the narrowing of the vessel lumen which is a consequence of

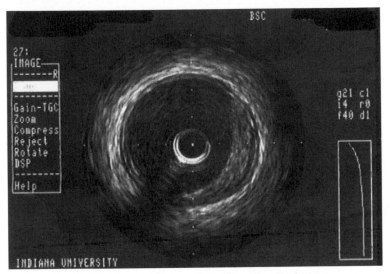

Fig. 3.1. Intravascular ultrasound image of an atherosclerotic plaque

the plaque, but occurs as a result of plaque rupture. Plaque rupture is related to the so-called stability or instability of the plaque. In addition to several other factors, plaque morphology is of primary importance in plaque rupture. A large lipid nucleus combined with a thin fibrous cap containing only a few SMCs has a greater tendency to rupture than a plaque consisting of a small nucleus and thick fibrous cap. Plaque rupture can lead to intramural bleeding, exposition of thrombogenic subendothelial structures (collagen, cholesterol ester, etc.) and to thrombosis (Fig. 3.2). Currently, there are numerous research projects underway investigating whether there are gender-related differences in plaque composition and in factors contributing to plaque rupture. It is being debated, for example, whether plaques with thin capsules occur more frequently in young women who suffer a myocardial infarction than in older women. Thus far, however, there are no clear results of this research.

In addition to the developments described above, inflammatory processes will cause a further progression of atherosclerosis. The individual steps of this process remain largely unexplained and are also the subject of intensive research. Important factors of this process are intercellu-

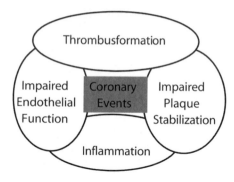

Fig. 3.2. Potential mechanisms for plaque instability and coronary events. (Modified from Koenig 2001)

lar adhesion molecules, cytokines, and other proteins occurring with inflammatory processes.

Female hormones influence the genesis and progression of atherosclerotic plaques as well as the inflammatory processes which lead to their progression.

Effects of Estrogen

Estrogens, in particular 17β-estradiol, have an effect not only on reproduction and the development of sexual organs, but also on many other biological structures and processes, especially the endothelium, lipid metabolism, and coagulatory system (Fig. 3.3). Because the incidence of CHD is negligible in premenopausal women without risk factors but increases significantly after menopause, estrogens were assumed to have a cardioprotective effect. This assumption was supported by the observation that estrogen replacement is connected with a decrease in many of the negative changes in risk profile connected with menopause (Nabulsi et al. 1993).

It has been previously hypothesized that the most important cardioprotective effect of estrogen was its effect on lipid metabolism; however, since observational studies demonstrated a reduction in cardiovascular mortality with estrogen replacement therapy even in women without dyslipidemia, this mechanism can only partially explain the assumed cardioprotective effect. Most likely, other effects are of greater importance, par-

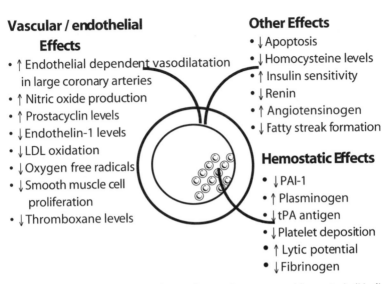

Vascular / endothelial Effects

- ↑ Endothelial dependent vasodilatation in large coronary arteries
- ↑ Nitric oxide production
- ↑ Prostacyclin levels
- ↓ Endothelin-1 levels
- ↓ LDL oxidation
- ↓ Oxygen free radicals
- ↓ Smooth muscle cell proliferation
- ↓ Thromboxane levels

Other Effects

- ↓ Apoptosis
- ↓ Homocysteine levels
- ↑ Insulin sensitivity
- ↓ Renin
- ↑ Angiotensinogen
- ↓ Fatty streak formation

Hemostatic Effects

- ↓ PAI-1
- ↑ Plasminogen
- ↓ tPA antigen
- ↓ Platelet deposition
- ↑ Lytic potential
- ↓ Fibrinogen

Fig. 3.3. Effects of estrogen on the cardiovascular system and hemostasis (Modified from Hayes 2000)

ticularly an improvement in endothelium-dependent vessel reactivity, decreased low-density lipoproteins (LDL) oxidation, decrease of the thrombotic potential, decreased expression of adhesion molecules, increased fibrinolytic activity, and increased glucose metabolism.

Effect of Estrogen on Vascular Reactivity and Endothelial Function

Atherosclerosis is associated with a decrease in vasodilation capacity combined with increased vasoconstriction due to neurohormonal stimulation. Numerous animal research studies and clinical trials have conclusively shown that estrogen is able to decrease arterial vascular tone and maintain the vasodilating capacity of the coronary arteries (Weiner et al. 1994; Wellman et al. 1996). For example, estrogen is able to abolish acetylcholine-induced vasoconstriction in atherosclerotic coronary arteries. (Collins et al. 1995). Since increased coronary vasoconstriction is of significant importance in the pathogenesis of unstable angina, myocardial in-

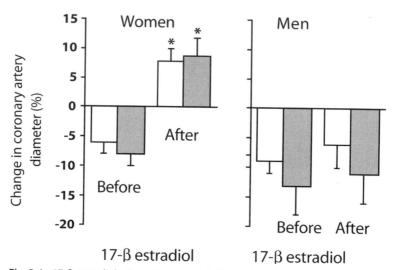

Fig. 3.4. 17-β estradiol attenuates acetylcholine-induced coronary arterial constriction in women but not in men. (From Collins et al. 1995)

farction, and sudden cardiac death, lowering of arterial vascular tone leads to a decrease in the incidence of vascular spasms and subsequently of ischemia. In addition, it has been hypothesized that fewer plaque ruptures occur as a result of the decreased vascular reactivity, thus slowing the progression of the coronary atherosclerosis (Williams et al. 1992, 1994); however, estrogen is not able to induce regression in plaque size. In addition, estrogen leads to a decreased production of endothelin-1, a strong vasoconstrictor, thus reducing ischemia as well.

On one hand, estrogen has a direct effect on the arterial wall primarily by blocking calcium channels, and on the other hand, it has an indirect and long-term effect by increasing expression of a large number of genes which play a key role in the regulation of arterial vessel resistance (e.g., prostacyclin, endothelin-1), in the repair of vessel injuries (e.g., epidermal growth factor, TGF-β) and in coagulation processes (e.g., fibrinogen, protein-S; Table 3.1). Long-term effects are facilitated by two different estrogen receptors (alpha and beta) which are located in the nucleus of vessel wall cells (in particular SMCs).

Estrogen causes increased production of nitrogen monoxide (NO),

Table 3.1. Effects of sex hormones on the arterial wall. (Modified from Knopp 1998)

	Estrogen	Estrogen + progesterone	Androgen
LDL penetration	↓	?	?
Vasodilatation	↑	↓	↑
Repair mechanisms	↓	↓/↑	No effect
Atherogenesis	↓	↓/↑	↑

LDL low-density lipoproteins

which, in addition to vessel dilation via relaxation of smooth muscle cells, has three or possibly four additional important cardioprotective benefits:

1. It reduces platelet adhesion and aggregation.
2. It has an anti-adrenergic effect which manifests itself in a reduced myocardial oxygen requirement.
3. It has an anti-oxidative effect since it is able to capture free radicals.
4. Potentially, an anti-arrhythmic effect. It remains to be seen, however, whether the suppression of ischemia-induced cardiac arrhythmias shown in animal experiments has any clinical correlation.

Effect of Estrogen on Lipid Metabolism

The lipid profile in healthy premenopausal women is cardioprotective: high high-density lipoproteins (HDL); low LDL; and low total cholesterol. With a decrease of endogenous estrogen production (either secondary to natural menopause, chemotherapy, or ovariectomy) a change from a more atherogenic pattern is observed with elevated cholesterol- and LDL levels and relatively low HDL (see also chap. 9).

Animal research data have shown that estrogen prevents the accumulation and hydrolysis of cholesterol in the arterial cell wall independently of plasma lipid levels (Haarbo et al. 1991).

Furthermore, estrogen supports the removal of lipoproteins through the liver, especially LDL. Because of increased expression of apolipopro-

Table 3.2. Effects of sex hormones on lipoprotein levels and lipoprotein metabolism. (Modified from Knopp 1998)

	Estrogen	Estrogen + progesterone	Androgen
Level			
Triglycerides	↑	=	↓
VLDL	↑	=	↓
LDL	↓	↑/↓	↑
HDL	↑	=	↓
Apo-1	↑	=	↓
Metabolism			
Cholesterol absorption	=	?	?
VLDL secretion	↑	↓	↓
LDL formation	↑	↑/?	?
LDL removal	↑	↓	↓
HDL transport	↑	↓	↓
Lp(a) concentration	↓	=	↓

VLDL very low-density lipoprotein, *LDL* low-density lipoprotein, *HDL* high-density lipoprotein, *Apo A-1* apoprotein A-1, *Lp(a)* Lipoprotein (a)

tein B/E receptors in the liver, there is also increased binding of these lipoproteins (Table 3.2).

Anti-oxidative Effect of Estrogen

Supraphysiological levels of 17-β estradiol inhibit LDL oxidation and the formation of cholesterol esters, thus leading to a protection of endothelial cells (Negre-Salvayre et al. 1993; Rifci et al. 1992).

Effect of Estrogen on Inflammation

Estrogen modulates immunological and inflammatory reactions during the genesis and progression of the atherosclerosis of coronary arteries. For example, it has been noted that it affects the expression of interleukin-1 and 6 (IL-1, IL-6), of monocyte chemotactic protein-1 (MCP-1), of growth factor A, of tumor necrosis factor alpha (TNF-a), and of the nuclear factor kappa B (NF-kB), a transcription factor that regulates the expression of many genes (see Register et al. 1995).

Effect of Estrogen on Hemostasis

Estrogen affects several antithrombotic factors, thereby counteracting thrombus formation after plaque erosion or rupture in the coronary artery. Estrogen lowers fibrinogen- and plasminogen activator inhibitor-1 (PAI-1) levels, thus leading to an increase in the fibrinolytic potential (Gebara et al. 1995; Meilahn et al. 1992). Since the Framingham study it has been known that elevated fibrinogen is an independent risk factor for fatal and nonfatal myocardial infarction. PAI-1 is an inhibitor of fibrinolysis. In addition, it has been demonstrated that estrogen lowers the rise in PAI-1 levels, especially in the morning. This counteracts the hypercoagulability known to be connected to time of day and the known rise in coronary events in the morning.

Estrogen causes an increase in plasminogen levels which also changes the equilibrium in the direction of fibrinolysis.

The effects of estrogen on the coagulation cascade is complex and depends on dosage and manner of administration (e.g., oral, transdermal). Most studies show that estrogen causes a minimal rise in the pro-coagulatory factor VII; however, the procoagulatory effect due to increased factor VII production is clinically not very significant, since simultaneously there is an increase in protein C that degrades factor V and lowers the fibrinogen level.

In addition to these effects, estrogen also lowers antithrombin III and causes transient increases in factor IX and X levels; however, it is not yet evident whether these changes in levels are clinically significant.

◗ Summary

Atherosclerosis of the coronary arteries is the underlying pathophysiological mechanism of CHD and is the same for both genders. Acute coronary syndromes as well as myocardial infarctions occur as the result of a ruptured plaque. Currently, differences between the genders in plaque composition and rupturing are under investigation. Female hormones influence the genesis and progression of atherosclerotic plaques as well as the inflammatory processes that lead to their progression. Whether anti-atherogenic or pro-inflammatory properties are balanced or will shift the balance in one direction has yet to be determined.

Estrogen has the following beneficial effects:
- It improves endothelium-dependent vessel reactivity.
- It lowers LDL oxidation.
- It decreases the thrombotic potential.
- It increases fibrinolytic activity.

References

Chang WC, Nakao J, Orimo H, Murota SI (1980) Stimulation of prostacyclin biosynthetic activity by estradiol in rat aortic smooth muscle cells in culture. Biochim Biophys Acta 619:107–118

Collins P, Rosano G, Sarrel PM et al. (1995) Estrogen attenuates acetylcholine-induced coronary arterial constriction in women but not in men with coronary heart disease. Circulation 92:24–30

Gebara OC, Mittleman MA, Sutherland P et al. (1995) Association between increased estrogen status and increased fibrinolytic potential in the Framingham Offspring Study. Circulation 91:1952–1956

Gilligan DM, Quyyumi AA, Cannon RO III (1994) Effects of physiological levels of estrogen on coronary vasomotor function in postmenopausal women. Circulation 89:2545–2551

Haarbo J, Leth-Espensen P, Stenders S et al. (1991) Estrogen monotherapy and combined estrogen-progestogen replacement therapy attenuate aortic accumulation of cholesterol in ovariectomized cholesterol-fed rabbits. J Clin Invest 87:1274–1279

Harder DR, Coulson PB (1979) Estrogen receptors and effects of estrogen on membrane electrical properties of coronary vascular smooth muscle. J Cell Physiol 100:375–382

Hayes SN (2000) Heart disease in women. In: Murphy JG (ed) Mayo clinical cardiology review. Williams & Wilkins, Lippincott, p 1122

Herrington DM (1991) Sex hormones and normal cardiovascular physiology in women. In: Burgess A (ed) Women and heart disease. Dunitz, London, pp 243–264

Jiang C, Sarrel PM, Lindsay DC, Poole-Wilson PA. Collins P (1991) Endothelium-independent relaxation of rabbit coronary arteries by 17-beta-estradiol in vitro. Br J Pharmacol 104:1033–1037

Jiang C, Sarrel PM, Poole-Wilson PA, Collins P (1992) Acute effect of 17-beta estradiol on rabbit coronary artery contractile responses to endothelin-1. Am J Physiol 263:H271–275

Kannel WB, Wolf PA, Castelli WP et al. (1987) Fibrinogen and the risk of cardiovascular disease. The Framingham Study. JAMA 258:1183–1186

Karas RH, Patterson BL, Mendelsohn ME (1994) Human vascular smooth muscle cells contain functional estrogen receptor. Circulation 89:1943–1950

Knopp RH (1998) Estrogen, female gender and heart disease. In: Topol EJ (ed) Textbook of cardiovascular medicine. Lippincott-Raven, Philadelphia/PA, p 207-208]

Koenig W (2001) Inflammation and coronary heart disease. Cardiol Rev 9:32

Losordo DW, Kearney M, Kim EA et al. (1994) Variable expression of the estrogen receptor in normal and atherosclerotic coronary arteries of premenopausal women. Circulation 89:1501–1510

Mendelsohn ME, Karas RH (1999) The protective effects of estrogen on the cardiovascular system. N Engl J Med 340:1801

Meilahn EN, Kuller LH, Matthews KA et al. (1992) Hemostatic factors according to menopausal status and use of hormone replacement therapy. Ann Epidemiol 2:445–455

Morales DE, McGowan KA, Grant DS et al. (1995) Estrogen promotes angiogenic activity in human umbilical vein endothelial cells in vitro and in a murine model. Circulation 91:755–763

Nabulsi AA, Folsom AR, White A et al. (1993) Association of hormone replacement therapy with various cardiovascular risk factors in postmenopausal women. N Engl J Med 2328:1069–1075

Negre-Salvayre A, Pieraggi MT, Mabile L et al. (1993) Protective effect of 17-beta estradiol against the cytotoxicity of minimally oxidized LDL to cultured bovine aortic endothelial cells. Atherosclerosis 99:207–217

Register TC, Bora TA, Adams MR (1995) Estrogen inhibits activation of arterial NF-kB transcription factor in early diet-induced atherogenesis. Abstract. Circulation 92:I-628

Regnstrom J, Nilsson J, Trovnvall P et al. (1992) Susceptibility to low-density lipoprotein oxidation and coronary atherosclerosis in man. Lancet 339:1183–1186

Rifci VA, Khachadurian AK (1992) The inhibition of low-density lipoprotein oxidation by 17-beta estradiol. Metabolism 41:1110–1114

Sudhir K, Chou TM, Mullen WL et al. (1992) Mechanism of estrogen-induced vasodilation: in vivo studies in canine coronary conductance and resistance arteries. J Am Coll Cardiol 20:452–427

The Writing Group for the PEPI Trial (1995) Effects of estrogen or estrogen/progestin regimens on heart disease risk factors in postmenopausal women. The Postmenopausal Estrogen/Progestin Interventions (PEPI) trial. JAMA 273:199–208

Venkov CD, Rankin AB, Vaughan DE. Identification of authentic estrogen receptor in cultured endothelial cells. Circulation 94:727–733

Weiner CP, Lizasoain I, Baylis SA et al. (1994) Induction of calcium-dependent nitric oxide synthases by sex hormones. Proc Natl Acad Sci USA 91:5212–5216

Weksler BB (1993) Hemostasis and thrombosis. In: Douglas PS (ed) Cardiovascular Health and Disease in Women. Saunders, Philadelphia, pp 231–251

Wellman GC, Bonev AD, Nelson MT et al. (1996) Gender differences in coronary artery diameter involve estrogen, nitric oxide, and Ca^{2+}-dependent K^+ channels. Circ Res 79:1024–1030

Williams JK, Adams MR, Herrington DM, Clarkson TB (1992) Short-term administration of estrogen and vascular responses of atherosclerotic coronary arteries. J Am Coll Cardiol 20:452–457

Williams JK, Honore EK, Washburn SA, Clarkson TB (1994) Effects of hormone replacement therapy on reactivity of artherosclerotic coronary arteries in cynomolgus monkeys. J Am Coll Cardiol 24:1757–1761

4

Stable Angina

Definition and Pathophysiology of Angina Pectoris . . . 48

Diagnosis Based on Symptoms 49

Diagnostic Evaluation 52

Medical Management 64

**Percutaneous Coronary Intervention
for Stable Angina** 67

References 77

Definition and Pathophysiology of Angina Pectoris

Angina is a clinically defined syndrome rather than a disease and does not always imply the presence of coronary artery disease; however, angina pectoris is the most common manifestation of coronary artery disease and in this situation symptoms are due to myocardial ischemia. The most frequent underlying cause is an atherosclerotic coronary artery stenosis causing an imbalance between oxygen demand and supply with either physical exertion or emotional stress. Either tachycardia, increased myocardial wall tension, increased myocardial contractility, or all of them are associated with higher oxygen requirements that cannot be met. Angina is less often due to increased vascular reactivity leading to vasospasm (i.e., Prinzmetal's angina) or endothelial dysfunction (i.e., syndrome X). There is not only a linear correlation between angina and the intensity of exercise, but symptoms are also reproducible. Symptoms due to chronic stable angina are usually relieved within 3 min of rest. Angina occurring at rest is not due to chronic stable angina, but due to vasospasm, an arrhythmia, or an acute coronary syndrome. Pain lasting longer than 30 min is very suggestive of myocardial infarction.

Typical angina is described as retrosternal heaviness, pressure, or squeezing sensation with radiation across the pericardium, up the neck or

Table 4.1. Angina pectoris classification by the Canadian Cardiovascular Society

I	No symptoms with ordinary physical activity, such as walking and climbing stairs. Angina with strenuous or rapid or prolonged exertion at work or recreation
II	Slight limitation of ordinary activity. Angina while walking more than two blocks on the level and climbing more than one flight of stairs at a normal pace. Angina in cold, in wind, or when under emotional stress, or only during the few hours of awakening
III	Marked limitation of ordinary physical activity. Angina while walking one to two blocks on the level and climbing more than one flight in normal conditions
IV	Inability to carry on any physical activity without discomfort. Angina at rest

down the ulnar surface of the left arm. The right arm, the shoulders, and the lateral aspects of both arms may be involved as well. Some patients describe a "strangling" or "suffocating" sensation. Frequently, the pain starts in the arm or neck and travels to the midsternal area. The chest discomfort may be associated with or overshadowed by dyspnea, extreme fatigue, lightheadedness, nausea, and/or epigastric discomfort.

The classification of angina pectoris by the Canadian Cardiovascular Society (CCS) into four categories based on functional capacity is given in Table 4.1.

Diagnosis Based on Symptoms

Diagnosis of CAD in women remains a challenge. Until recently gender differences in clinical presentation were not appreciated. It was assumed that angina in men and women was similar if not equal; however, women have a high likelihood of atypical symptoms such as dyspnea without pain or chest discomfort, indigestion, pain between the shoulder blades, or retrosternal burning. Not infrequently extreme fatigue, new onset of reduced exercise capacity, or epigastric discomfort are the only clinical findings suggestive of CAD. Atypical angina is most common in elderly women. In addition, women have a higher prevalence of rest pain and symptoms induced by emotional stress (De Sanctis 1993).

Data from the Framingham Heart Study demonstrated that women develop angina approximately 10 years later in life than men. Women 75 years or older have angina more than men of similar age. Based on these findings and the fact that in the past most studies were conducted in middle-aged men and women it has become clear that the medical literature reports a prevalence of angina in women not higher than 50 %. Early gender-specific data from the Framingham Heart Study as well showed that more women than men without coronary artery lesions have angina (65 vs 37 %). Subsequently women had a lower likelihood of cardiac events on followup. That led to the false assumption that angina is a relatively benign condition in women and does not need medical attention; however, the prognosis of stable CAD is similar for men and women and with a combined annual death rate and myocardial infarction rate of 2–3 % is quite good.

It cannot be stressed often enough that diagnosis of CAD in women with angina is a difficult task, even further complicated by the mispercep-

Table 4.2. Pretest likelihood of coronary artery disease in symptomatic patients according to age and gender (in percent). (Adapted from Recommendations of the Task Force of the European Society of Cardiology 1997, and Del Valle et al. 1999)

Age (years)	Typical angina Women	Men	Atypical angina Women	Men	Nonanginal pain Women	Men
30–39	26	70	4	22	1	5
40–49	55	87	13	46	3	14
50–59	79	92	32	59	8	22
60–69	90	94	54	67	19	28

tion by the woman herself and health care providers that CAD is a man's disease. A possible approach to diagnosis (and management) is the combined evaluation of pain character and numbers of risk factors: Women with several risk factors (including menopause) and typical angina have a high likelihood of CAD (80–90 %). In contrast, the likelihood of CAD in premenopausal women with atypical symptoms and no cardiovascular risk factors is generally low (<4 %).

The following approach is helpful to determine the pretest likelihood of coronary heart disease (CHD) in women. If a woman is premenopausal and is not diabetic, the likelihood of coronary disease is very low; however, the risk of coronary disease in a diabetic woman, independent of menopausal status, does not differ from that in men. The likelihood of coronary disease in postmenopausal women depends on the number of risk factors (with diabetes the most important one) and the character of chest pain. The more risk factors and the more typical the chest pain, the higher the likelihood of disease.

Table 4.2 shows average pretest likelihoods of CHD in women with typical and atypical symptoms.

Prinzmetal's or Variant Angina

Vasospastic or Prinzmetal's angina is caused by vasospasm. Arteriosclerotic plaques represent predilection sites; however, vasospasms may also occur in normal coronary arteries. The right coronary artery is affected more frequently than the left. Women suffer more frequently from vasospastic angina than men. Young female smokers and women with migraines or Raynaud's phenomenon are affected in particular. Cocaine abuse also leads to vasospasm. Thrombus formation with subsequent infarction development is possible, since vasospasm leads to intermittent hemostasis. The pain of Prinzmetal's angina occurs predominantly at rest and is associated with ST-segment elevation in the ECG and occasionally with cardiac arrhythmias. Aside from giving up smoking and cocaine abuse, calcium channel blockers are the therapy of choice. The long-term prognosis is excellent (5-year survival rate of 97 %).

Syndrome X

Syndrome X describes the simultaneous presence of exertional angina pectoris, an abnormal stress test, and angiographically normal coronary arteries. This syndrome is encountered in women more frequently than in men. More than 50 % of women with syndrome X are premenopausal. Less than 50 % of these women have typical symptoms. The underlying cause is endothelial dysfunction and probably also reduced vasodilatory capacity in the microcirculation. The long-term prognosis is excellent and does not differ from that of healthy women of similar age. Calcium channel blockers are the most therapeutically effective medications, but pain is often difficult to influence and is often associated with a considerable reduction in quality of life.

◉ Summary

Diagnosis of CAD in women remains a challenge, even after a detailed history and thorough physical examination. Women present with a high incidence of atypical symptoms. It is not uncommon for symptoms such as dyspnea, sensation of epigastric fullness, retrosternal burning and easy fatigability to be angina equivalents. This is particularly true for elderly women. This picture is complicated by the observation that even women with angiographically normal coronary arteries frequently experience angina. If risk factors are present (menopause and diabetes mellitus are the most significant risk factors), a proven practical approach has been to maintain a high level of suspicion until the diagnosis of CHD has been unequivocally excluded.

Diagnostic Evaluation

Accurate and timely diagnosis is an indispensable prerequisite in reducing morbidity and mortality of CHD. Aside from a careful history, including an evaluation of risk factors, and a thorough physical exam, electrocardiogram and stress testing make up the fundamental diagnostic methods. Examination via cardiac catheterization is the final link in the chain of diagnostic modalities. Numerous studies have shown gender differences in the predictive value of these methods; therefore, knowledge of these differences is necessary for the optimal application of these tests.

Electrocardiogram

The resting ECG has only limited sensitivity in the diagnosis of CHD. More than 30 % of all patients with stable angina have a normal ECG. On the other hand, 32 % of all women who do not have CHD, but who do have angina, exhibit nonspecific repolarization abnormalities (as opposed to only 23 % of all men). The presence of Q-waves is associated with a high specificity for a prior myocardial infarction; however, the sensitivity is low.

Stress Testing, Including Stress Echocardiography and Nuclear Imaging

Determination of Pretest Probability for CHD

The principles of non-invasive diagnostic tests are the same for men and women (Lualdi et al. 1997); however, non-invasive tests are generally less reliable in women than in men due to the fact that the modalities available to us were predominantly validated in trials conducted in middle-aged men. Upon careful selection and interpretation of different stress tests, it is nevertheless possible to draw conclusions regarding the presence and severity of CHD.

The decision on whether a particular test is indicated in the presumptive diagnosis of CHD should be based on a fundamental understanding of the methods available and on Bayes' Theorem, which states that the post-test likelihood of disease depends on pretest likelihood, test accuracy, and test results. The predictive accuracy of a test is related to disease prevalence in the population studied. In other words, women with a low probability of CHD (so-called pretest probability) continue to have a low probability of CHD even in light of a positive test result. In cases of high probability, the probability remains high even if the result is negative (Seafstreom 1998). Therefore, routine testing of asymptomatic patients should be avoided. Stress tests are appropriate for those patients with an intermediate probability of CHD, e.g., patients with atypical symptoms and multiple risk factors, or patients with typical symptoms but lack of risk factors (Redberg 1998). In all other cases, a stress test is not indicated, e.g., in young premenopausal women with no risk factors who exhibit atypical symptoms, or in older women with risk factors and typical angina. In the latter case a cardiac catheterization without prior non-invasive evaluation is appropriate.

Selection of Stress Test

Stress test selection depends upon whether the patient is able to exercise to her target heart rate, whether there are resting ECG changes, and upon comorbidities (e.g., asthma, obesity, medication). For example, severe arthritis or deconditioning may result in an adequate exercise study.

An exercise stress test is principally preferable to a pharmacological stress test, since physical exertion most closely reflects physiological conditions and allows conclusions to be drawn relative to daily activities; however, the prerequisite is that the woman be able to achieve 85 % of maximum predicted heart rate (220 minus patient's age). A pharmacological stress test is indicated in all other cases.

The following stress tests are available:
1. Exercise electrocardiogram
2. Stress scintigram (thallium-201 or technetium-99)
3. Stress echocardiogram

Items 2 and 3 may be carried out in conjunction with exercise, as well as in conjunction with pharmacological provocation with dobutamine, dipyridamole, or adenosine.

Stress ECG

A stress ECG is of limited value in women. It is associated with a higher rate of false-positive results in women (38–67 %) than in men (7–44 %). On the other hand, false-negative results are less common in women

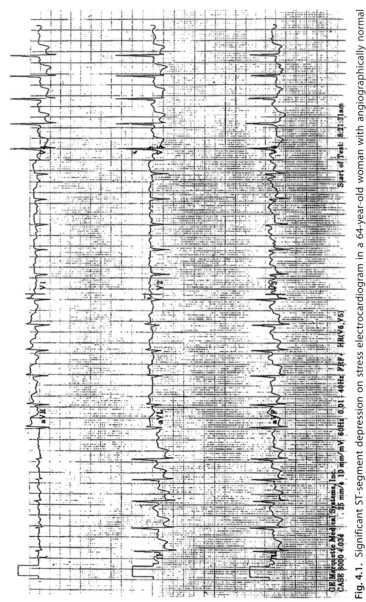

Fig. 4.1. Significant ST-segment depression on stress electrocardiogram in a 64-year-old woman with angiographically normal coronary arteries

(12–22 %) than in men (12–40 %), despite the fact that factors which favor the likelihood of false-negative results (greater prevalence of single-vessel disease, reduced exercise tolerance) are more often present in women (Alexander et al. 1998). The CHD may therefore be excluded with relative certainty if the stress ECG is normal, but caution is warranted if pathological findings are present. In the latter case the use of another non-invasive test (e.g., stress echocardiography) is indicated. Gender-specific meta-analyses on stress ECGs come to the conclusion that sensitivity and specificity of stress ECGs are lower in women than in men (Kwok et al. 1999). In 21,667 men, the sensitivity of the stress ECG was 68 % and the specificity 77 %. In 3721 women the sensitivity was 61 % and the specificity 70 % (Gianrossi et al. 1999). Multiple factors play a role in the gender differences:

1. Women have a high prevalence of nonspecific ST–T wave changes, which increases the likelihood of false-positive results.
2. For reasons not yet clarified and independent of age, women develop ECG changes with stress that have a negative impact on the interpretation of the stress ECG (a digoxin-like effect of estrogen has been discussed).
3. The pretest probability of CHD is low in young women, likewise coupled with the risk of a high rate of false-positive test results.

Caution is therefore required in the interpretation of positive-stress ECGs. In order to increase diagnostic accuracy, an exercise stress test should be performed in conjunction with an imaging technique (either echocardiogram or scintigram; Fleischmann et al. 1998; Kwok et al. 1999), in particular in women with atypical symptoms or the absence of risk factors. Although a negative stress ECG does not absolutely rule out CHD, it is associated with a good prognosis.

An example of a false-positive stress ECG is shown in Fig. 4.1.

Nuclear Imaging

Nuclear isotopes can be used to assess myocardial perfusion and regional blood flow. The most commonly used isotopes are thallium-201 and technetium-99, either in form of technetium-99 sestamibi (Cardiolite) or in form of technetium-99m tetrofosmin (Myoview). Isotopes are taken up by myocytes in proportion to blood flow, which presumes the presence of viable myocardial cells. Decreased blood flow leads to reduced uptake that is reflected in a perfusion defect. The defect is called "reversible" if the area shows re-uptake in the resting state; hence, no necrotic tissue is present.

Images are either obtained in the form of a planar scintigram or via single photon emission computed tomography (SPECT), which is generally preferable to planar scintigraphy, since SPECT is associated with less interference from non-cardiac structures and SPECT is able to detect even small areas of hypoperfusion (Fintel et al. 1989).

Nuclear imaging in both men and women is associated with a higher sensitivity and specificity in comparison with conventional-exercise ECG. Despite this, gender differences continue to be present.

Meta-analyses of stress tests in women *using thallium-201* revealed a moderate increase of sensitivity and specificity in comparison with exercise ECG, but both parameters were still reduced in comparison with those of men (Hansen et al. 1996). In particular, the specificity was lower in women than in men (sensitivity in women 78 vs 84 % in men; specificity in women 64 vs 87 % in men; Kwok et al. 1999). The frequent occurrence of breast attenuation artifacts is the most common reason for the reduced specificity. Since thallium-201 is a relatively low-energy isotope, it can lead to an apparently reduced image of the anterior and anterolateral wall in women.

Nuclear imaging studies with technetium-99 Sestamibi are associated with a higher specificity than studies with thallium-201. Technetium-99 is a relatively high-energy isotope and therefore leads to fewer breast artifacts. Taillefer et al. (1997) reported a 25 % increase in test specificity with technetium-99m sestamibi over thallium-201 in women. The sensitivity and specificity with technetium-99m was 72 and 86 %, respectively, and the sensitivity and specificity of the thallium investigation was 75 and 62 %, respectively.

Stress Echocardiography

Stress echocardiography has two advantages over nuclear imaging techniques: (a) it can be carried out by a cardiologist in the office; and (b) it is not associated with radiation exposure. It can be combined with exercise (treadmill or bicycle stress test) or with pharmacological stressors. The most commonly used agents are dobutamine, arbutamine, dipyridamole, and adenosine. Dobutamine is utilized most frequently. Supine bicycle stress testing is the method of choice since images can be obtained at peak exercise and the increased preload during stress further increases sensitivity and test accuracy. With treadmill stress testing imaging is done with the patient in the supine position immediately after exercise. Image acquisition should occur within 1 min, requiring excellent and experienced op-

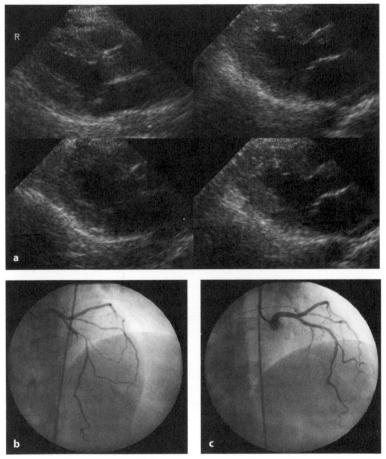

Fig. 4.2a–c. Abnormal stress. Echocardiogram in a 67-year-old woman. Stress-induced hypokinesis of the interventricular septum (parasternal long axis). The coronary angiogram revealed a high-grade left anterior descending artery (LAD) lesion that was successfully treated with balloon angioplasty and stent implantation

erators. Only high-quality images permit reliable interpretation. Presently, all images are stored digitally, thereby allowing side-by-side assessment of the echocardiogram before and after exercise. Four different planes are obtained: parasternal long and short axes and apical four- and two-chamber view. Sixteen segments of the left ventricle are examined for wall motion abnormalities pre- and post test. Ischemia is present if exercise causes hypokinesis or akinesis in one or more ventricular segments. Localization of the ischemia allows conclusions to be drawn as to which coronary vessel exhibits stenosis.

Stress echocardiography is the only non-invasive stress test without gender differences in sensitivity and specificity. Marwick et al. (1995) found a sensitivity of 85 and a specificity of 77 % for both men and women. A recently published meta-analysis confirmed these data. In this publication the sensitivity of stress electrocardiography in women was 86 % and the specificity 79 % (Sawada 1998). Aside from the excellent accuracy of the method, stress echocardiography is also the most economical test. Unnecessary coronary angiography or other non-invasive tests can be avoided if stress echocardiography is the first one utilized in the workup of a presumptive diagnosis of CHD in women. Stress echocardiography is able to categorize a woman at intermediate risk for CHD to either the high-risk or low-risk group. In addition, the stress echocardiography provides insights into ventricular function, wall thickness, and valvular disease.

Figure 4.2 shows a stress echocardiogram of a 67-year-old woman with stress-induced wall motion abnormalities of the septum.

Pharmacological Stress Tests

Non-invasive tests using pharmacological agents (either vasodilators or positive inotropic agents) are employed in patients who are unable to perform adequate exercise or if the target heart rate cannot be achieved. All pharmacological stress tests have to be combined with an image modality (either nuclear perfusion imaging or echocardiography). Pharmacological stress tests play a more important role for women than for men, since women less frequently than men achieve the target heart rate necessary for meaningful interpretation of the stress test. Dobutamine is the most often used stressor. It is a sympathomimetic agent and thus increases myocardial contractility, heart rate, and ultimately oxygen consumption. Marwick et al. (1995) and Secknus et al. (1997) demonstrated that there are basically no gender differences in the physiological effects of dobutamine; however, an increase in heart rate occurs more rapidly in women than in men. In women, sensitivity and specificity of stress echocardiography with dobutamine is slightly less than with physical stress. Despite these limitations, stress echocardiography remains the method of choice for women.

The most commonly used vasodilators are dipyridamole and adenosine. The major mechanism of action is through an increase in coronary blood flow within the normal vascular bed (as much as fourfold) and hence through a reduced perfusion in stenotic sections (so-called coronary steal phenomenon). They produce numerous side effects (e.g., facial redness, headache, dyspnea, hypotension) and are contraindicated in case of asthma or obstructive pulmonary disease.

⊙ Summary

Non-invasive diagnostic tests are only meaningful if the physician is able to determine the pretest probability of CHD on the basis of medical history and physical examination, and then to compare the pretest probability with the results of a carefully selected stress test (Fig. 4.3; Table 4.3). The predictive value of a stress ECG is low and often associated with false-positive test results if not combined with an imaging technique. Despite the high initial costs, stress echocardiography is the most accurate and most economical stress test for women. It is therefore the method of choice; however, stress echocardiography requires imaging by experienced and technically well-versed operators. If this is not possible, a technetium-99 sestamibi SPECT is the best alternative with a sensitivity similar to, but a specificity lower than, stress echocardiography. Radiation exposure is a further disadvantage of nuclear stress testing.

Stress tests are contraindicated in women with unstable angina. After myocardial infarction, a stress test should not be performed earlier than 3 days after the event.

Table 4.3. Average sensitivity and specificity of various exercise stress test modalities in the diagnosis of coronary artery disease in women. (Modified from Kwok et al. 1999, and Douglas 2001)

Exercise test	No. of women	Sensitivity (%)	Specificity (%)
ECG	3721	61	70
Thallium	842	78	64
Echo	296	86	79

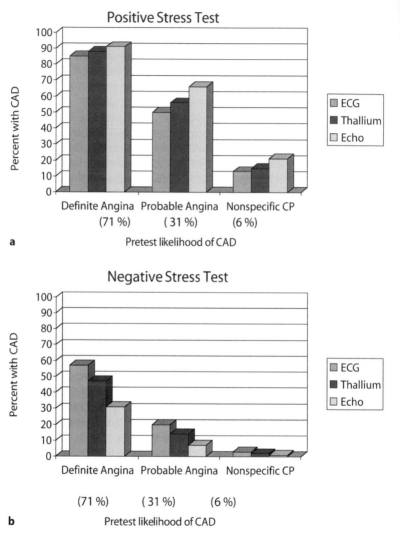

Fig. 4.3 a, b. Posttest likelihood of coronary artery disease (*CAD*) in a 55-year-old woman, depending on pretest probability of disease, type of chest pain (*CP*), and test results

Electron Beam Computed Tomography

Electron beam computed tomography (EBCT) assesses the extent of coronary artery calcification as a marker of atherosclerosis. Calcium scores are based on the degree and density of calcifications. The detection of calcium by EBCT has good sensitivity for the diagnosis of coronary artery stenoses, ranging from 85 to 100 %; however, the specificity for significant lesions is low and varies from 41 to 76 %. Accuracy in men and women seems to be similar. The clinical value of EBCT is still unclear. The ACC/AHA Expert Consensus Document on EBCT did not recommend it for the diagnosis of CHD. Given the high likelihood of false-positive results, it may lead to additional and unnecessary testing.

Magnetic Resonance Imaging

Magnetic resonance imaging (MRI) has high spatial resolution capability, allowing excellent image quality in both genders. In contrast to nuclear imaging, no breast attenuation artifacts occur. Based on these facts, it can be assumed that no gender differences are present. Thus far, however, no gender-specific studies are available to answer this question. Evaluation of myocardial perfusion is also possible if the MRI is carried out with a contrast agent (e.g., gadolinium). Based on basic research data MRI holds promise for noninvasively imaging plaque composition and eventually vulnerable plaques. In addition, MRI is able to noninvasively reconstruct coronary anatomy and thus to provide a noninvasive coronary angiogram. Magnetic resonance angiography even allows for visualization of arterial blood flow without administration of a contrast agent.

Diagnostic Cardiac Catheterization

Few data exist on gender differences and diagnostic cardiac catheterization. Steen et al. (1992) found a higher rate of vascular complications as well as a higher percentage of women who develop renal insufficiency. The smaller body size, older age of the women at the time of presentation, and the increased prevalence of diabetes mellitus play an important role. Other complications, including myocardial infarction, stroke, and death, occurred at equal frequency in both genders.

Table 4.4. Value of diagnostic tools for the detection of coronary artery disease in women (0 to ++++). (Adapted from Patterson 1997)

	R or R+S	False (+)	False (−)	Nondiag-nostic	Vali-dation	Risk	Costs
ECG	R	+++	++	+++	+++	++	++
SPECT	R/S	++	+	++	+++	++	+++
ECHO	R/S	++	+	++	++	++	+++
PET	R/S	+	+	+	++	++	++++
MRI	R/S	++	+	++	+	++	++++
EBCT	R	++	+	+	++	0	++
CA	R	0	0	0	++++	++++	++++

R rest, *S* stress, *SPECT* single photon emission computed tomography with thallium-201 or technetium-99m sestamibi, *ECHO* echocardiogram, *PET* positron emission tomography, *MRT* magnetic resonance imaging, *EBCT* electron-beam computed tomography, *CA* coronary angiography

The accuracy of the various diagnostic tests in women are listed in Table 4.4.

Gender Differences in the Use of Diagnostic Cardiac Catheterizations and Percutaneous Coronary Intervention

Studies from the mid-1980s demonstrated that men are six times more likely to undergo cardiac catheterization than women. Invasive diagnostic procedures were performed to a lesser extent in women than in men even after a positive stress test or in women with unstable angina. Gender differences in clinical care have certainly diminished in recent years, but full equality still does not exist (Table 4.5). Even after an abnormal nuclear stress imaging study, only 34 % of women, but 45 % of men, undergo coronary angiography. The Worcester Heart Attack Study shows similar data for patients with a myocardial infarction; men were 1.69 times more likely than women to be referred for a cardiac catheterization, despite recurrent

Table 4.5. Frequency of coronary angiography (*CA*) by gender in patients with stable angina pectoris

Authors	Year	No. of patients	CA in women (%)	CA in men (%)
Tobin et al.	1987	390	5	34
Ayanian and Epstein	1991	49623	16	28
Chae et al.	1993	840	34	45
Morise et al.	1994	1980	24	21
Shaw	1994	840	34	45
Gregor et al.	1994	9737	18	24

angina and functional disability from their symptoms. Numerous factors have been cited to account for the observed gender differences in the referral rate for coronary angiography. One possible explanation is the still widespread (and incorrect) assumption that angina pectoris in women is associated with a better prognosis than in men. The older age of the women and the higher incidence of comorbidities in women at the time of initial CHD manifestation may play a role as well.

Gender bias in referral for angiography cannot be excluded as well. On the other hand, any perceived gender bias in referral patterns could reflect an inappropriate overuse of diagnostic cardiac catheterizations in men at low risk for cardiac events.

However, after a diagnostic cardiac catheterization has been performed, the number of women who will undergo a subsequent revascularization procedure [either coronary artery bypass graft or percutaneous coronary intervention (PCI)] does not differ essentially from that of men (Bell et al. 1993). Although men are slightly more likely to have bypass surgery than women, the proportion of women referred for PCI is higher than that of men. Weintraub et al. and the Asymptomatic Cardiac Ischemia Pilot (ACIP) Study, which conducted a gender-specific subgroup analysis, came to the same conclusion (Frishman et al. 1998). In contrast to these observations, more recent studies found no significant gender differences in referral patterns.

There is no doubt that an early invasive diagnostic evaluation with subsequent revascularization in patients at high or intermediate risk for further cardiac events is associated with a better prognosis, independent of gender. Moreover, it could be shown that women who do not undergo early and aggressive work-up and therapy, but are merely treated medically, have an even worse prognosis than men. Given these facts, only early diagnosis of CHD, including cardiac catheterization and early aggressive treatment including revascularization, will reduce morbidity and mortality of CHD in women.

Medical Management

Optimal therapy for stable angina pectoris includes the following:
- Non-pharmaceutical measures (weight loss, quitting smoking, healthy diet)
- Modification of risk factors (lipid reduction, regulation of blood pressure and diabetes, aspirin, physical activity)
- The intake of antianginal medications (i.e., nitrates and beta-blockers)

Few studies have examined gender differences with respect to medical therapy of stable CHD. Most likely there are differences in efficacy, bioavailability, side effects, and toxicity of the various drugs based on hormonal status, distribution of body fat, weight, and generally higher age of women at the time of manifestation of CHD; however, a recently published review on this topic found that medical therapy equally benefited men and women (Fig. 4.4.).

Beta-blockers

Beta-blockers are the cornerstone for medical therapy not only for stable angina, but also for acute coronary syndromes and acute myocardial infarction. Preference should be given to beta-blockers with predominant inhibition of myocardial β_1-receptors (metoprolol, atenolol, esmolol).

The therapeutic goal is a heart rate of 50–60 beats/min. Contraindications include second- or third-degree arteriovenous blockage, heart rate

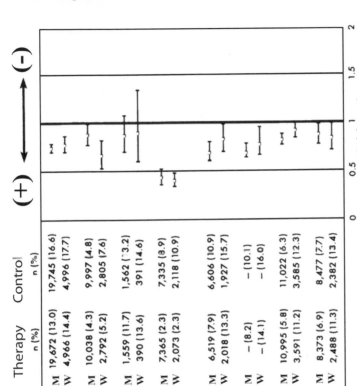

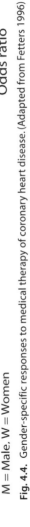

		Therapy n (%)	Control n (%)
Platelet inhibitors	M	19,672 (13.0)	19,745 (16.6)
	W	4,966 (14.4)	4,996 (17.7)
Beta-Blocker	M	10,038 (4.3)	9,997 (4.8)
	W	2,792 (5.2)	2,805 (7.6)
Calcium Channel- Blocker	M	1,559 (11.7)	1,562 (13.2)
	W	390 (13.6)	391 (14.6)
Nitroglycerin	M	7,365 (2.3)	7,335 (8.9)
	W	2,073 (2.3)	2,118 (10.9)
Thrombolysis	M	6,519 (7.9)	6,606 (10.9)
	W	2,018 (13.3)	1,927 (15.7)
Fibrinolytic Agents	M	– (8.2)	– (10.1)
	W	– (14.1)	– (16.0)
Comparative trials	M	10,995 (5.8)	11,022 (6.3)
	W	3,591 (11.2)	3,585 (12.3)
ACE-Inhibitors	M	8,373 (6.9)	8,477 (7.7)
	W	2,488 (11.3)	2,382 (13.4)

M = Male, W = Women

Fig. 4.4. Gender-specific responses to medical therapy of coronary heart disease. (Adapted from Fetters 1996)

below 60 beats/min, blood pressure below 90 mmHg, decompensated heart failure, and obstructive lung disease. The presence of emphysema or asthma alone (no active bronchospasm!) is only a relative contraindication. Equivalent doses of beta-blockers lead to higher plasma levels in women than in men, possibly via gender differences in the cytochrome P450 system and hence to different hepatic metabolization of the drug (Walle et al. 1989; Gilmore et al. 1992). Based on multiple studies this seems to be the only gender difference.

Nitrates

After conversion to "nitric oxide," nitrates lead to dilatation of arteries, arterioles, and veins. Venous dilatation reduces preload and pulmonary capillary pressure; arterial vasodilatation reduces blood pressure, total vascular resistance, and afterload. Moreover, nitrates lead to both dilatation of normal and arteriosclerotic coronary arteries and thereby to increased coronary blood flow. Isosorbide dinitrate and isosorbide mononitrate are available in multiple formulations with short and long half-lives. To avoid tolerance, it is important to maintain a nitrate-free interval over several hours/day. Although nitrates are very effective in alleviation of angina pectoris, as yet no studies have demonstrated a mortality benefit. Studies examining gender differences do not exist (Abrams 1997).

Calcium Channel Blockers

Calcium channel blockers inhibit calcium entry into smooth muscle cells, myocardial cells, and in the cardiac conductive system. They lead to vasodilatation including the coronary arteries, to reduced myocardial contractility and heart rate, and consequently to reduced oxygen consumption in the myocardium and increased coronary perfusion (Frishman 1997). Indeed, all three classes of calcium channel blockers (dihydropyridines such as nifedipine and amlodipine, phenylalkylamines such as verapamil, and diltiazem) are effective in the treatment of angina pectoris. In contrast to beta-blockers, however, calcium channel blockers have not been shown to reduce mortality after myocardial infarction. Some studies report a reduction in reinfarction for long-acting calcium channel blockers (e.g., slow-release forms of verapamil or diltiazem). Short-acting calci-

um channel blockers, however, are associated with a higher rate of myocardial infarction in men and in women. In the Nurses Health Study
women who took calcium channel blockers for blood pressure control
were at higher risk for myocardial infarction or sudden cardiac death
compared with women who took other anti-hypertensive medications
(Michels 1998). Verapamil clearance is increased in women compared
with men because of a higher activity of the cytochrome P 450 system.
Amlodipine leads to a more rapid reduction in blood pressure in women
than in men (Kloner et al. 1996).

⊘ Summary

Beta-blockers and nitrates (along with aspirin) are first-line medications for
women with angina. Calcium channel blockers (preferable verapamil or
diltiazem) should only be used if beta-blockers are contraindicated and
should only be administered in long-acting form.

Percutaneous Coronary Intervention for Stable Angina

Unfortunately, a systematic investigation of gender differences with respect to success and complication rates of percutaneous transluminal
coronary angioplasty (PTCA) and other forms of PCI does not exist. Even
those large studies that compared multivessel angioplasty with bypass
surgery only rarely conducted gender-specific subgroup analyses. The fact
remains that at the time of CHD manifestation, on average, women are
older and have more comorbidities than men. This constellation has a
negative effect on morbidity and mortality with coronary intervention.
On the other hand, the hormonal status may have a positive impact on
success rate; however, as long as no specific literature exists to answer this
question, our knowledge must be restricted to the limited number of
works available.

Primary angioplasty for acute myocardial infarction and in comparison with thrombolytic therapy is discussed in Chap. 5, and glycoprotein
IIb/IIIa receptor antagonists is discussed in Chap. 6.

Since 1977, when the first balloon dilatation was performed by Gru-
entzig at the University of Zurich, there has been a tremendous progress
in PCIs, and consequently, the number of procedures (as well as indications) has steadily increased.

A particular increase occurred with the introduction of stents by Sigwart in 1987. Presently, stents are used in 80 % of cases given the lower risk of abrupt vessel closure and the reduced restenosis rate. Worldwide, the number of annual PTCAs exceeds 1 million.

The underlying mechanism of PTCA is complex, but it consists mainly of two components: firstly, in fracture of the atheromatous plaque, which involves localized intramural dissection; and secondly, in an expansion of the non-atheromatous portions of the vessel.

The most important complications following PTCA and stent implantation are abrupt vessel closure from extensive dissection, a "no-reflow" phenomenon from distal embolization of plaque material or thrombus (particularly in degenerated venous bypass grafts or in patients with angiographically visible thrombus), and restenosis. Prior to the availability of stents, abrupt vessel closure was the most feared complication and occurred in approximately 7 % of all coronary interventions. It was the leading cause of myocardial infarction, death, or need for emergency bypass surgery due to PTCA. Presently, the incidence of abrupt vessel closure has been reduced to less than 1 %. The death rate with coronary intervention, on average, does not exceed 0.5 %. Myocardial infarctions are either caused by abrupt vessel closure (i.e., in case of a significant dissection) or by distal embolization. In the latter case, most periprocedural myocardial infarctions are non-ST-segment-elevation myocardial infarctions. They occur in approximately 4 %. The incidence of Q-wave infarction is much less and, on average, less than 1 %. Vascular complications are more common with coronary intervention than with a diagnostic cardiac catheterization. They occur in 5–9 % of cases (Popma et al. 1993).

Besides improved operator experience and advancements in technology, the use of potent platelet inhibitors (ASA, ticlopidine, clopidogrel, GP IIb/IIIa receptor antagonists) further reduces the risk or complications in coronary interventions (see Chap. 6).

Clinical factors that increase the mortality risk from abrupt vessel closure include reduced ventricular function, advanced age, and dilatation of an artery that supplies a large area of viable heart muscle.

The following patient characteristics (a) and angiographic findings (b) are associated with an increased risk of abrupt vessel closure:
a) ▪ multivessel disease
   ▪ acute coronary syndromes
b) ▪ angulation (>90)
   ▪ tortuous artery

- complete occlusion
- long (>10 mm) stenosis
- calcifications
- ostial stenoses
- stenoses with inclusion of large side branches
- bifurcation lesions
- angiographically visible thrombus
- venous bypass stenoses

The ACC/AHA classification of coronary artery stenoses with respect to success and complication rates and indications for other interventional procedures are in cardiology textbooks.

Gender-Specific Success and Complication Rates for Balloon Angioplasty

During the past decade there has been considerable interest and controversy with respect to the importance of gender in contributing to mortality and complication rate after PCI. Most registries from the 1980s and early 1990s comparing gender-related differences in outcomes after balloon angioplasty (stents and other devices for coronary intervention were not available then) have shown significantly higher in-hospital mortality rate, a higher complication rate, and a lower success rate in women than in men.

The National Heart, Lung and Blood Institute (NHLBI) 1985–1986 PTCA Registry reported a significantly higher rate of death, dissection, abrupt vessel closure, vasospasm, and ventricular fibrillation in women, and a procedural success rate of only 70 %. (Presently, success rates have improved for both men and women and are reported to be 95 % or higher for both genders; see Table 4.6.). The increased mortality in women could partially be explained by the older age and higher incidence of cardiovascular risk factors, especially diabetes and hypertension; however even after adjustment for these variables female gender was still an independent predictor of death.

The researchers investigated whether the smaller body surface area, a surrogate for small vessel size in women, may have played a significant role. But re-analysis of the same NHLBI Registry data revealed no correlation between body weight, body surface area, body mass index, and mortality in female patients. (It is now well known that independent of gender, complications with coronary interventions occur more often in individuals of smaller body size.) The registry found that women were more susceptible to dissection, and when acute vessel closure occurred, women were more likely to die. The reasons still remain unclear. Women may have different autonomic and hemodynamic responses to acute vessel closure than men. This hypothesis is substantiated by the observation that women are more likely to become hypotensive and bradycardic after abrupt closure; however, there are most likely differences between men and women that are not known and that have not been incorporated in multivariate analyses.

In contrast to the NHLBI registry, in a study by Malenka et al. (1999) and another study by Weintraub et al. (1994) gender was not an independent risk factor for in-hospital mortality. Although the reported in-hospital mortality rate for women undergoing balloon angioplasty was higher than that for men (1.6 vs 0.7 %, and 0.7 vs 0.1 %, respectively), and women had a higher rate of emergency bypass surgery (2.6 vs 2.0 %), after statistical adjustment for age, risk factors, history of myocardial infarction, and unstable angina there was no gender difference. In these registries the higher complication rate with coronary intervention could be attributed to the older age of the women at the time of hospital admission and the higher incidence of comorbidities (see Table 4.6).

To elucidate the reasons for the higher in-hospital mortality in women Welty et al. (2001) prospectively analyzed the outcome of almost 6000 angioplasties (2000 in women, 60 % unstable angina) between 1989 and 1995 with respect to the timing of complications. They looked at three different time frames: the time of the intervention; the first 24 h after intervention; and the time from day 1 until discharge. In-laboratory complications at the time of balloon angioplasty were essentially the same for men and women. All differences did not reach statistical significance. Within the first 24 h, however, women had a higher risk of hypotension and in particular vascular complications (1.6 vs 0.6 %); however, the most striking difference was in the time frame from 24 h after the procedure and either death or discharge. Twenty-four hours after the procedure, women had a significantly higher mortality rate (1.2 vs 0.52 %). In further analysis of these data they found that two-thirds of the excess mortality was due to non-cardiac but procedure-related complications, in particular renal failure and vascular complications including bleeding, hypotension, and stroke.

Table 4.6. Gender differences in angiographic success rate and mortality of elective coronary angioplasty. (Adapted from Douglas 2001)

Authors	Period	Angiographic success (%)		Mortality (%)	
		Women	Men	Women	Men
Cowley et al. (1985)	1978–1982	60	66	1.7	0.3
Kelsey et al. (1993)	1985–1986	84	87	2.6	0.3
Arnol et al. (1994)	1980–1988	94	93	1.1	0.3
Bell et al. (1993)	1988–1990	87	90	2.9	1.4
Weintraub et al. (1996)	1980–1991	91	90	0.7	0.1
O'Connor et al. (1999)	1994–1996			1.3	0.9

In contrast to deaths of women, deaths among men were primarily cardiac in nature. Welty et al. (2001) concluded that the complications probably are avoidable if operators would pay more attention to contrast load (in particular in diabetic women), sheath size, management of vascular access site after sheath removal, and anticoagulation regimens. It is noteworthy that there were no significant gender differences in cardiac complications such as need for bypass surgery or incidence of myocardial infarction.

Besides renal failure and, to a lesser extent, stroke, the most important gender difference with respect to in-hospital mortality is the rate of vascular complications, even in the most recent years. Despite smaller sheath size and use of smaller devices, all recent studies report a higher incidence of groin complications. The smaller artery size and smaller body surface area play an important role, but most of the reasons have not yet been clarified.

Gender-Specific Success and Complication Rates for Coronary Intervention with Stent Implantation

Since the mid-1990s coronary stenting has become the mainstay of catheter-based interventions in both genders. Balloon angioplasty alone (without stent) and atherectomy procedures significantly decreased in those years. Presently, approximately 80 % of all PCIs in the United States are performed with implantation of a stent; however, despite a dramatic increase in stent usage, no large study exists to provide insights into gender-specific differences following stent implantation.

The few available data report a lower complication- and death-rate compared with balloon angioplasty, but still a higher mortality and complication rate in women than in men.

Peterson et al. (2001) evaluated data from the National Cardiovascular Network (NCN) Database from 1994 to 1998 with respect to gender and with respect to device used. Thirty-three percent of the 110,000 patients were women. Stents were used in 37 % of women and 40 % of men. Eight percent of patients presented with acute myocardial infarction. Procedural success was approximately 90 % in both genders; however, women still had a higher in-hospital mortality after stent implantation than men, even after adjustment for differences in baseline characteristics (relative risk 1.07). In addition – as importantly as mortality – despite the fact that overall complications were low, women were nearly twice as likely to have a stroke (0.4 vs 0.2 %), a Q-wave myocardial infarction (odds ratio 1.28), or vascular complications (odds ratio 2.09). Stroke and vascular complications were significantly higher in women than in men even after adjustment for baseline characteristics and age. In-hospital mortality never equalized between men and women, although the gender gap narrowed once clinical factors were considered.

Data from the Health Care Cost and Utilization project in approximately 70,000 patients with stent placement, of whom 36 % were women, show that women still had a twofold higher mortality than men (Watanabe et al. 2001). This was true for patients with and without myocardial infarction. Similarly, the need for emergency bypass surgery was higher in women than in men, although this finding did not reach statistical significance in patients with acute myocardial infarction. This study demonstrates that despite improved overall outcomes in patients receiving stents, women still do worse than men.

A small study from Spain from 1997 came to the same short-term results (Alfonso et al. 2000). After stent placement, women had a higher in-hospital mortality than men (3.6 vs 0.8 %); however, despite poorer initial results, the event-free survival and restenosis rate after 2 years was not different between men and women, even in patients who initially had no procedural success.

Ahmed et al. (2001) examined the effect of gender on early and 1-year clinical outcomes in patients undergoing stent implantation in saphenous vein graft lesions from 1994 to 1998. Despite a similar procedural success between men and women, women had a higher in-hospital and 30-day mortality (3.2 vs 1.6 %, and 4.4 vs 1.9 %, respectively). This increased risk was independent of body mass index, body surface area, and other confounding factors; however, mortality did not differ after 1 year. In addition to a higher early mortality, women had a higher incidence of vascular complications (only 6 % GP IIa/IIIb) requiring surgical repair (12 vs 7.3 %).

Figure 4.5 shows a successful angioplasty with stent implantation in a 92-year-old woman.

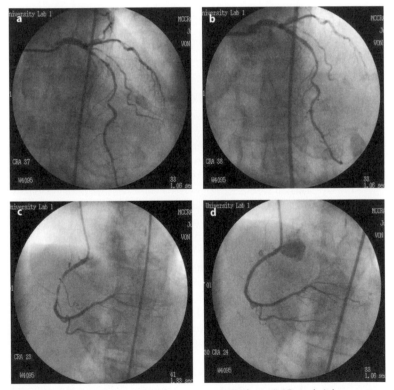

Fig. 4.5a–d. Successful two-vessel coronary angioplasty (LAD and right coronary artery) in a 92-year-old woman with angina class III according to classification of Canadian Cardiovascular Society

⊘ **Summary**

Despite recent refinements in techniques in PCI and better adjunctive therapy, women continue to be at higher risk than men for complications after PCI and continue to have a higher in-hospital mortality, regardless of the device technology used.

Restenosis

Gender is not a risk factor for restenosis. In the Multihospital Eastern Atlantic Restenosis Trial Study, which was conducted just a few years ago, the rate of *angiographic* restenosis was 39 % in men and 42 % in women. A carefully executed meta-analysis of 31 reliable studies (of 212 published) found that female gender had no influence on restenosis rate (Bobbio et al. 1991).

Rotablator Therapy, Directional Coronary Atherectomy, Laser Therapy

Alternative techniques to balloon angioplasty and stent implantation are used in those patients whose lesion characteristics make a satisfactory result with conventional interventional therapy unlikely. These lesions include highly calcified stenoses, long diffuse stenoses, and ostial stenoses. The limited indication classifies these procedures as "niche procedures." They are used in approximately 5 % of all coronary interventions, both in the United States and in Europe. With the exception of rotablator therapy, which is the most adequate therapy for highly calcified lesions, a worldwide decline of these alternative techniques has been noted.

Atherectomy requires the use of larger guide catheters and correspondingly larger introducer sheaths than plain balloon angioplasty, thus increasing the risk of peripheral and coronary artery injuries. As expected, the complication rate reported for these new devices is also higher in women (who generally have smaller arteries) than in men. A success rate of 89 % in women vs 95 % in men is reported for directional atherectomy. The risk of procedure-related myocardial infarction is 5 and 4 %, respectively. Peripheral vascular complications, emergency bypass surgery, and in-hospital mortality are also more common in women.

The Percutaneous Excimer Laser Coronary Angioplasty Registry found a higher incidence of perforations in women and particularly in diabetic women (Bell et al. 1994; Casale et al. 1993; Fishman et al. 1992); however, laser treatment is rarely used.

Multivessel Coronary Intervention – When PCI?
When Bypass Surgery? Comparison in Randomized Studies

Women with left main disease, multivessel disease involving the left anterior descending artery, and/or reduced left ventricular systolic function (particularly diabetic women) still benefit most from coronary artery bypass surgery in comparison with PCI; however, this viewpoint may change in the near future. Aside from these high-risk patients, at least 50 % of women are candidates for both PCI as well as for bypass surgery. The question arises as to whether gender differences exist favoring one method over the other.

Percutaneous coronary intervention has been compared with bypass surgery in eight randomized studies since 1992. Only 15–27 % of all patients included were women; hence, no subgroup analysis was possible given the low number of cases. The Bypass and Angioplasty Revascularization (BARI) Study included enough women but did not perform a subgroup analysis (Pocock et al. 1995). Unfortunately, no gender-specific meta-analysis of all eight studies exists to date. A gender-independent meta-analysis of all available data unanimously comes to the conclusion that neither PCI is superior to bypass surgery, and vice versa. Long-term outcome is similar for both methods and both genders. All patients, whether man or woman, had a lower risk for in-hospital complications. In BARI, deaths occurred in 1.3 % of the bypass patients and in 1.1 % of the angioplasty patients, strokes in 0.8 and 0.2 %, respectively, and myocardial infarction (Q-wave infarction) in 4.6 and 2.1 %, respectively. Patients who underwent angioplasty, however, had a higher incidence of angina in the first years after the intervention, most likely secondary to incomplete revascularization. After 3 years, this difference disappeared. After 5 years, 8 % of the bypass patients needed a repeat revascularization procedure compared with 54 % of the angioplasty patients, given the high risk of restenosis with balloon angioplasty. Long-term survival rates were excellent in both groups: 90 % of all patients were still alive after 3 years and 80 % after 6 years (Fig. 4.6.). When it is considered that women were old-

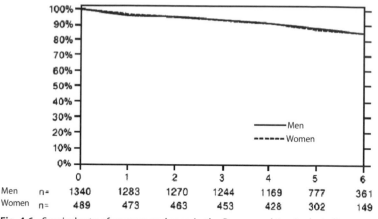

Fig. 4.6. Survival rate of women and men in the Bypass and Angioplasty Revascularization Study (1996)

er at the time of surgery and had more comorbidities than men, they actually demonstrated a better clinical outcome than men.

The only exception were diabetic patients with multivessel disease. Based on a subgroup analysis from the BARI study, the 5-year survival rate for diabetics who underwent bypass surgery (independent of gender) was higher than that for diabetics who underwent angioplasty.

It has to be kept in mind that these data were derived in an era prior to the development of glycoprotein IIb/IIIa receptor antagonists and the widespread use of stents. In anticipation of further significant improvements, not only in the field of interventional cardiology but also with coronary bypass surgery (e.g., rapamycin-coated stents and less invasive surgical methods such as surgery on a beating heart), it has become clear that these data are already outdated.

⊗ Summary

Long-term outcome for women who are candidates for either coronary angioplasty or bypass surgery is excellent independent of choice of procedure and gender. Due to a higher likelihood of incomplete revascularization with PCI, patients who undergo coronary intervention experience more angina in the first 3 years after the intervention and more frequently require a second procedure (in most cases a second PCI) than coronary artery bypass patients; however, women undergoing PCI have a lower risk of a periprocedural Q-wave infarction. In addition, the procedure is less invasive.

References

Abrams J (1997) The organic nitrates and nitroprusside. In: Frishman WH, Sonnenblick EH (eds) Cardiovascular Pharmacotherapeutics. McGraw-Hill, New York, pp 253–265

Ahmed JM, Dangas G, Lansky AJ et al. (2001) Influence of gender on early and one-year clinical outcomes after saphenous vein graft stenting. Am J Cardiol 87:401–405

ACIP Investigators (1992) Asymptomatic cardiac ischemia pilot (ACIP) study. Am J Cardiol 70:744–747

Alexander KP, Shaw LJ, Delong ER et al. (1998) Value of exercise treadmill testing in women. J Am Coll Cardiol 32:1657

Alfonso F, Hernandez R, Banuelos C et al. (2000) Initial results and long-term clinical and angiographic outcome of coronary stenting in women. Am J Cardiol 86:1380–1383, A5

Arnold AM, Mick MJ, Piedmonte MR, Simpfendorfer C (1994) Gender differences for coronary angioplasty. Am J Cardiol 74:18

Ayanian JZ, Epstein AM (1991) Differences in the use of procedures between women and men hospitalized for coronary artery disease. N Engl J Med 325:221–225

BARI-Studie (1996) Comparison of coronary bypass surgery with angioplasty in patients with multivessel disease. The Bypass Angioplasty Revascularization Investigation (BARI-) Investigators. N Engl J Med 335:217-225]

Bell MR, Holmes DR, Berger PB et al. (1993) The changing in-hospitl mortality of women undergoing percutaneous transluminal coronary angioplasty. JAMA 269:2091

Bell MR, Garratt KN, Bresnahan JF, Holmes DR jr (1994) Immediate and long-term outcome after directional coronary atherectomy: analysis of gender differences. Mayo Clin Proc 69:723–729

Bell MR, Berger PB, Holmes DR jr, Mullany CJ, Bailey KR, Gersh BJ (1995) Referral for coronary artery revascularization procedures after diagnostic coronary angiography: evidence for gender bias? J Am Coll Cardiol 25:1650–1655

Bobbio M, Detrano R, Colombo A et al. (1991) Restenosis rate after percutaneous transluminal coronary angioplasty: A literature overview. J Invas Cardiol 3:214–224

Casale PN, Whitlow PL, Franco I et al. (1993) Comparison of major complication rates with new atherectomy devices for percutaneous coronary intervention in women versus men. Am J Cardiol 71:1221–1223

Chae SC, Heo J, Iskandrian AS et al. (1993) Identification of extensive coronary artery disease in women by exercise single-photon-emission computed tomographic (SPECT) thallium imaging. J Am Coll Cardiol 21:1305–1311

Chiriboga DE (1993) A community wide perspective of gender differences and temporal trends in the use of diagnostic and revascularization procedures for acute myocardial infarctions. Am J Cardiol 71:268–273

Cowley MJ, Mullin SM, Kelsey SF et al. (1985) Sex differences in early and long-term results of coronary angioplasty in the NHLBI PTCA registry. Circulation 71:90

Chronos NA, Ewing HL, McGorisk GM et al. (1997) Percutaneous transluminal coronary angioplasty in women. In: Julian DG, Wegner NK (eds) Women and heart disease. Mosby, St. Louis/MO, p 183–192

Del Valle M, Frishman WH, Charney P (1999) In: Charney P (ed) Coronary artery disease in women. American College of Physician Press, Philadelphia, p 37

De Sanctis RW (1993) Clinical manifestations of coronary artery disease: Chest pain in women. In: Wenger NK, Speroff L, Packard B (eds) Cardiovascular health and disease in women. Le Jacq Communications, Greewich/CT, p 67

Douglas PS (2001) Coronary artery disease in women. In: Braunwald E, Zipes DP und Libby P (eds) Heart disease. Saunders, Philadelphia, vol. 58, p 2045]

Fetters JK, Peterson ED, Shaw LJ et al. (1996) Sex-specific differences in coronary artery disease risk factors, evaluation, and treatment: Have they been adequately evaluated? Am Heart J 131:796–804

Fintel DJ, Links JM, Brinker JA et al. (1989) Improved diagnostic performance of exercise thallium-201 single photon emission computed tomography over planar imaging in the diagnosis of coronary artery disease: A receiver operating characteristic analysis. J Am Coll Cardiol 13:600

Frishman WH, Gomberg-Maitland M, Hirsch H et al. (1998) Differences between male and female patients with regard to baseline demographics and clinical outcomes in the Asymptomatic Cardiac Ischemia Pilot (ACIP) Trial. Clin Cardiol 21:184–190

Fishman RF, Friedrich SP, Gordon PC et al. (1992) Acute and long-term results of new coronary interventions in women and the elderly. Circulation 86 (Suppl 1): I-255

Fleischmann KE, Hunink MGM, Kunts KM, Douglas PS (1998) Exercise echocardiography or exercise SPECT imaging? A meta-analysis of diagnostic test performance. JAMA 280:913

Frishman WH (1997) Calcium-channell blockers. In: Frishman WH, Sonnenblick EH (eds) Cardiovascular Pharmacothereutics. McGraw-Hill, New York, pp 101-130

Frishman WH, Gomberg-Maitland M, Hirsch H et al. (1998) Differences between male and female patients with regard to baseline demographics and clinical outcomes in the Asymptomatic Cardiac Ischemia Pilot (ACIP) Trial. Clin Cardiol 21:184–190

Gianrossi R, Detrano R, Mulvihill D et al. (1999) Exercise-induced ST depression in the diagnosis of coronary artery disease in women. Am J Cardiol 83(5):660–666

Gilmore DA, Gal J, Gerber JG, Nies AS (1992) Age and gender influence the stereo-selective pharmacokinetics of propranolol. J Pharm Exp Ther 261:1181–1186

Gregor RD, Bata I, Eastwood BJ et al. (1994) Gender differences in the presentation, treatment, and short-term mortality of acute chest pain. Clin Invest Med 17:551–562

Hansen CL, Crabbe D, Rubin S (1996) Lower diagnostic accuracy of tallium-201 SPECT myocardial perfusion imaging in women: an effect of smaller chamber size. J Am Coll Cardiol 28(5):1214–1219

Kelsey SF, James M, Holubkov AL et al. (1993) Results of percutaneous transluminal coronary angioplasty in women: 1985–1986 NHLBI coronary angioplasty registry. Circulation 87:720

Kloner RA, Sowers JR, DiBona GF et al. (1996) Sex- and age-related antihypertensive effects of Amlodipine: the Amlodipine Cardiovascular Community Trial Study Group. Am J Cardiol 77:713–722

Kwok Y, KIM C, Grady D et al. (1999) Meta-analysis of exercise testing to detect coronary artery disease in women. Am J Cardiol 83:660

Lualdi JC, Douglas PS (1997) Echocardiography for the assessment of myocardial viability. J Am Soc Echocardiogr 10:772–780

Malenka DJ, O'Rourke D, Miller MA et al. (1999) Cause of in-hospital death in 12,232 consecutive patients undergoing percutaneous transluminal coronary angioplasty. Am Heart J 137;632

Marwick TH, Anderson T, Williams MJ et al. (1995) Exercise echocardiography is an accurate and cost effective technique for detection of coronary artery disease in women. J Am Coll Cardiol 26:335

Michels KB, Rosner BA, Manson JE et al. (1998) Prospective study of calcium-channel blocker use, cardiovascular disease, and total mortality among hypertensive women: the Nurses Health Study. Circulation 97:1540–1548

Morise AP, Singh P, Duval R (1994) Correlation of reported exercise test results with recommendations for coronary angiography in men and women with suspected coronary artery disease. Am J Cardiol 75:180–187

Neuhaus KL (1996) Qualitätssicherung bei Kroronararteriendilatation. Deutsch Aerztebl 51:3383–3385

O'Connor GT, Malenka DJ, Quinton H et al. (1999) Multivariate prediction of in-hospital mortality after percutaneous coronary interventions in 1994–1996. J Am Coll Cardiol34:681

Patterson RE (1997) Special problems with cardiovascular imaging to assess coronary artery disease in women. In: Julian DG, Wenger NK (eds) Women and heart disease. Dunitz, London, vol 6, p 95]

Peterson ED, Lansky AJ, Kramer J et al. (2001) Effect of gender on the outcomes of contemporary percutaneous coronary intervention. Am J Cardiol 88:359–364

Pocock SJ, Henderson RA, Rickards AF et al. (1995) Meta-analysis of randomised trials comparing coronary angioplasty with bypass surgery. Lancet 346:1184–1189

Popma JJ, Satler LF, Pichard AD et al. (1993) Vascular complications after balloon and new device angioplasty. Circulation 88:1569–1578

Recommendations of the Task Force of the European Society of Cardiology (1997) Management of stable angina pectoris. Eur Heart J 18:398

Redberg RF (1998) Diagnostic testing for coronary artery disease in women and gender differences in referral for revascularization. Cardiol Clin 16(1):67–77

Sawada SG (1998) Diagnostic and prognostic value of stress echocardiography (review). Cardiol Rev 6(2):96–99

Schulman KA, Berlin JA, Harless W et al. (1999) The effect of race and sex on physicians' recommendations for cardiac catheterization. N Engl J Med 340:618

Seafstreom K, Nielsen NE, Bjeorkholm A et al. (1998) Unstable coronary artery disease in post-menopausal women: identifying patients with significant coronary artery disease by basic clinical parameters and exercise test. IRIS Study Group. Eur Heart J 19(6):899–907

Secknus MA, Marwick TH (1997) Influence of gender on physiologic response and accuracy of Dobutamine echocardiography. Am J Cardiol 80(6):721–724

Shaw LJ, Miller DD, Romeis JC et al. (1994) Gender differences in the noninvasive evaluation and management of patients with suspected coronary artery disease. Ann Intern Med 120:559–566

Shaw LJ, Miller DD, Romeis JC et al. (1991) Gender differences in the noninvasive evaluation and management of patients with suspected coronary artery disease. Ann Intern Med 120:559

Steen MK, Jacobs AK, Freney D et al. (1992) Gender related differences in complications during coronary angiography. Circulation 86(Suppl I):254

Steingart RM, Packer M, Hamm P et al. (1991) Sex differences in the management of coronary artery disease. N Engl J Med 325:226–230

Taillefer R, DePuey EG, Udelson JE et al. (1997) Comparative diagnostic accuracy of Tl-201 and Tc-99 m sestamibi SPECT imaging (perfusion and ECG-gated SPECT) in detecting coronary artery disease in women. J Am Coll Cardiol 29:69

Tobin JN, Wassertheil-Smoller S, Wexler JP et al. (1987) Sex bias in considering coronary bypass surgery. Ann Intern Med 107:19–25

Walle T, Wall UK, Cowart TD, Conradi EC (1989) Pathway selective sex differences in the metabolic clearance of propranolol in human subjects. Clin Pramacol Ther46:257–263

Watanabe CT, Maynard C, Ritchie JL (2001) Comparison of short-term outcomes following coronary artery stenting in men versus women. Am J Cardiol 88:848–852

Weiner DA, Ryan TJ, Parsons L et al. (1995) Long-term prognostic value of exercise testing in men and women from the coronary artery surgery study (CASS) registry. Am J Cardiol 75:865

Weintraub WS, Wenger NK, Kosinski AS et al. (1994) Percutaneous transluminal coronary angioplasty in women compared with men. J Am Coll Cardiol 24:81

Weintraub WS, Kosinski AS, Wenger NK (1996) Is there a bias against performing coronary revascularization in women? Am J Cardiol 78:1154–1160

Welty FK, Lewis SM, Kowalker W, Shubrooks SJ Jr (2001) Reasons for higher in-hospital mortality >24 hours after percutaneous transluminal coronary angioplasty in women compared with men. Am J Cardiol 88:473–477

Wenger NK (1990) Gender, coronary artery disease, and bypass surgery. Ann Intern Med 112:557–558

5

Acute Myocardial Infarction

**Progression from Stable Coronary Heart Disease
to Myocardial Infarction** 84

Epidemiology of Acute Myocardial Infarction 85

Pathophysiology 87

Clinical Presentation of Acute Myocardial Infarction . . 89

**Criteria for the Diagnosis
of Acute Myocardial Infarction** 90

Therapy 92

Complications 101

Prognosis 102

**Influence of Gender on the Referral
for Coronary Angiography in Patients
with Acute Myocardial Infarction** 107

References 109

Progression from Stable Coronary Heart Disease to Myocardial Infarction

There is a gradual transition from stable to unstable angina and subsequently to myocardial infarction.

Chronic (stable) angina is most commonly due to a high-grade obstruction of the coronary arteries by atherosclerotic plaque. Progression to partial or complete mechanical obstruction – in other words, to non-Q-wave or Q-wave myocardial infarction – is unpredictable. In the presence of collaterals complete coronary artery occlusion may not lead to a myocardial infarction.

Rupture or erosion of an atherosclerotic plaque (most commonly in lesions <50 % in diameter) with superimposed nonocclusive thrombus is by far the most common cause of unstable angina. Only if myocardial necrosis occurs (determined by a rise in troponin T or I) is the patient classified as having a non-Q-wave myocardial infarction. The more recent terminology for a non-Q-wave myocardial infarction is non-ST-segment elevation myocardial infarction (NSTEMI). Given the fact that the underlying pathophysiology in unstable angina and NSTEMI is the same, they are frequently classified as acute coronary syndrome, which is the focus of Chap. 6.

Myocardial infarction in women differs from that in men on many levels:

- Epidemiology
- Clinical presentation
- Complication
- Response to treatment
- In-hospital and late mortality

These gender-related differences are poorly understood. Biological differences, particularly hormonal status, have been discussed; however, the fact that women with myocardial infarction tend to have a greater number of individual cardiovascular risk factors than men, present at least a decade later with their first myocardial infarction than men, and have a greater burden of comorbidities, may play a role as well. Studies are underway to elucidate these discrepancies.

Epidemiology of Acute Myocardial Infarction

Women who develop a myocardial infarction are approximately 20 years older than men; therefore, acute myocardial infarction is a disease of elderly women. After age 75 years, more women than men die from myocardial infarction. This can be explained by the fact that women live approximately 7–8 years longer than men and hence there is a greater representation of women in the elderly age group; however, mortality rates of 100,000 are still higher in men than in women.

Whereas by age 60 years 1 in 5 American men has had a coronary event, this occurs in only 1 of 17 American women (Fig. 5.1). This difference is less pronounced after age 75 years, but gender differences do not disappear completely.

Despite the fact that myocardial infarction is predominantly a disease of elderly women, there is an increase in the incidence of myocardial infarction in young women (<45 years). This tendency is especially striking in women with low socioeconomic status and consequently multiple cardiovascular risk factors. Presently, it is not uncommon to encounter a 40-

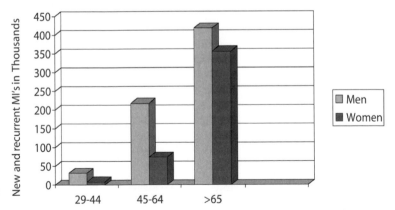

Fig. 5.1. Estimated annual number of myocardial infarctions in the United States in 1999 by age and gender. Data do not include silent myocardial infarctions. (Adapted from Heart and Stroke Statistical Update 1999. American Heart Association, Dallas, 1998, vol. 11)

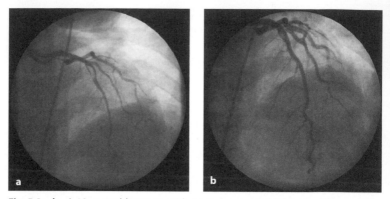

Fig. 5.2a, b. A 33-year-old woman with acute myocardial infarction. The coronary angiogram revealed a significant left anterior descending (LAD) artery lesion with thrombus. Patient was successfully treated with coronary angioplasty and stent implantation

year-old woman with an acute myocardial infarction. Figure 5.2 shows a significant left anterior descending artery lesion with thrombus formation in a 33-year-old premenopausal woman who presented with an acute anterior myocardial infarction.

Women suffering from an acute myocardial infarction are likely to be older and more likely to have multiple cardiovascular risk factors; however, women are less likely to be smokers than men. There is a high incidence of diabetes mellitus in women with myocardial infarction. The high prevalence of cardiovascular risk factors and comorbidities are in part due to the older age of women at the time of their first myocardial infarction.

Myocardial infarction is less often the first manifestation of coronary heart disease in women than it is in men (29 % in women vs 43 % in men). Angina pectoris is the most likely initial presentation of coronary artery disease in women; however, a significantly higher percentage of men presenting with angina subsequently develop a myocardial infarction, which has led to the erroneous conclusion that angina symptoms are less worrisome in women than in men.

Although the incidence of myocardial infarction has been steadily decreasing since the mid-1960s, this trend is less pronounced in women than in men. The reasons are uncertain. Several factors seem to play a role, including more preventive care in men than in women, increasing incidence of smoking in women, and the fact that women are still underdiagnosed and undertreated.

Pathophysiology

Based on the evolution of the pattern on the electrocardiogram (ECG) over several days, acute myocardial infarction patients are typically divided into those suffering a Q-wave or a non-Q-wave myocardial infarction (Table 5.1). Given the fact that Q waves frequently do not develop before several hours or days after a myocardial infarction, and not all patient with ST-segment elevation myocardial infarction ultimately develop Q waves on their ECG, a more recent nomenclature of acute myocardial infarction differentiates between ST-segment elevation myocardial infarction (STEMI; previous Q-wave myocardial infarction) and non-ST-segment elevation myocardial infarction (NSTEMI; previous non-Q-wave myocardial infarction). In both cases the underlying pathophysiology is the same. Endothelial injury, usually at sites of atherosclerotic plaque, and plaque ulceration or fissuring lead to platelet adhesion and aggregation, vasospasm, and eventually thrombus formation. Complete occlusion of the coronary artery results in STEMI, partial occlusion to a NSTEMI (Libby 1995); however, 40 % of all known NSTEMI are associated with complete occlusion of the coronary arteries as well.

There is no close correlation between severity of coronary artery lesion and the likelihood of a myocardial infarction. Most important is the morphology and composition of the atherosclerotic plaque. A meta-analysis of four studies has demonstrated that most (68 %) sites where myocardial infarction subsequently occurred showed less than 50 % stenosis on prior coronary angiograms. Only 14 % of infarcts were caused by stenosis greater than 70 %. These data demonstrate that not only localization and severity of coronary artery lesions denote adverse prognosis, but also plaque morphology. Diagnostic tools which are able to determine composition may play an important role in the future. Preliminary data are available for MRI and intravascular ultrasound.

Most likely there are no gender differences in the pathophysiological mechanism of an acute myocardial infarction; however, gender differences in the myocardial response to myocardial injury have been dis-

Table 5.1. World Health Organization criteria for diagnosis of acute myocardial infarction and differences between ST-elevation myocardial infarction (*STEMI*) and non-ST-elevation myocardial infarction (*NSTEMI*)

STEMI	NSTEMI
Chest pain or typical symptoms >30 min	Chest pain or typical symptoms >30 min
ST elevation of at least 1 mm in two consecutive leads or new left bundle branch block	ST depression or T-wave inversion
Positive myocardial enzymes	Positive myocardial enzymes
Thrombus rich in erythrocytes and fibrin	Thrombus rich in platelets
More common in men	More common in women

GUSTO Global Utilization of Streptokinase and Tissue Plasminogen Activator for Occluded Coronary Arteries, *TAMI* Thrombolysis and Angioplasty in Myocardial Infarction

cussed. For example, basic research data demonstrates that ion channels that are critically involved in the development of necrosis are differently expressed in men and women. It is unknown whether gender differences exist in atherosclerotic plaque composition and triggers of plaque rupture. Animal research data and clinical data from the National Registry of Myocardial Infarction Study (NRMI) suggest an interaction between estrogen and atherosclerosis. The pathophysiology of a myocardial infarction in a young woman (<45 years) may be different than the pathophysiology in elderly women.

Patients with NSTEMI in general have less obstructive thrombi which are constituted by less robust fibrin formation and a greater proportion of platelet aggregates. Patients with STEMI generally show an erythrocyte and fibrin-rich thrombus (Fuster et al. 1992). This distinction plays an important role with respect to therapy.

The incidence of NSTEMI is higher in women (25 %) than in men (16 %) (Hochman et al. 1997; see Table 5.1). This correlates well with findings that women appear to have a greater platelet reactivity compared with men.

Several factors determine the severity of a myocardial infarction:
- Localization of coronary artery occlusion (proximal or distal, major coronary artery or side branch)
- Extent of collateral circulation
- Metabolic activity of ischemic myocardium

The degree of hemodynamic impairment following acute myocardial infarction is related to the amount of myocardial damage (acute and chronic) and other factors such as valve dysfunction. Large myocardial infarctions are associated with decreased stroke volume and cardiac output and elevated left ventricular and diastolic pressure (LVEDP). Increased preload leads to left ventricular dilatation.

Clinical Presentation of Acute Myocardial Infarction

Silent Myocardial Infarction

In the Framingham Heart Study women had a higher proportion of silent myocardial infarction than men (Kannel et al. 1979; Murabito et al. 1993). The reasons remain unclear. Several factors may play a role. Women still consider coronary heart disease and in particular myocardial infarction as a "men's disease." Both older age and diabetes mellitus increase the likelihood of silent or unrecognized myocardial infarction. Atypical symptoms not only tend to delay presentation to the hospital but also to delay both diagnosis and subsequent treatment. In addition, despite the fact that women may perceive their pain in the setting of an acute myocardial infarction as abnormal, they tend to not acknowledge its serious nature until self-treatment and coping mechanisms fail. Impaired cognitive function in elderly women may play a role as well. In light of this data, improvement of therapy of myocardial infarction appears less important than prevention and change of societal and, in particular, female awareness.

Symptomatic Myocardial Infarction

Women seek medical attention for symptoms of acute myocardial infarction on average 1 h later then men, independent of age or social economic status (Meischke et al. 1993; Gurwitz et al. 1997). Initiation of treatment is longer as well (1.2 vs 1.0 h). The high incidence of atypical symptoms in women, in particular a higher incidence of abdominal discomfort, severe dyspnea, and marked weakness or frank syncope, may account for this treatment delay.

Late arrival to the hospital in the setting of an acute myocardial infarction and delay in therapy makes women less often eligible for thrombolytic therapy and is detrimental to myocardial salvage and subsequently detrimental to prognosis.

Criteria for the Diagnosis of Acute Myocardial Infarction

According to the World Health Organization (WHO), diagnosis of acute myocardial infarction requires at least two of the following three factors:
- Typical symptoms of myocardial ischemia of more than 30 min
- Evolutionary changes on serially obtained ECG tracings
- Increased levels of serum cardiac biomarkers

There are no gender differences in the objective diagnosis of STEMI; however all three components are present in only 50 % of patients – in both men and women.

Furthermore, ST-segment elevation and Q waves on the ECG, two features that are highly indicative of acute myocardial infarction, are seen in only 50 % of patients as well; hence, diagnosis of myocardial infarction may be difficult.

Clinical Presentation

Typical symptoms of myocardial infarction include substernal chest pressure with radiation to the left arm or neck, frequently associated with diaphoresis, nausea, vomiting, and/or shortness of breath. Only 25 % of women with acute myocardial infarction present with these symptoms;

25 % complain of indigestion or burning discomfort only. Another 25 % of women present with pain in the arm, neck, jaw, or back as their only symptom. The remainder of female patients are truly asymptomatic and are unable to recall any symptoms. In elderly women acute myocardial infarction is frequently solely manifested by shortness of breath, marked weakness, or frank syncope.

It cannot be stressed strongly enough that women present with atypical symptoms. Furthermore, symptoms may have already disappeared by the time the physician encounters the patient. If cardiovascular risk factors are present, a high level of suspicion should be maintained.

Electrocardiogram

Although the ECG is the most commonly used diagnostic tool for the recognition of acute myocardial infarction, the sensitivity does not exceed 50 %; hence, despite general agreement on ECG and vector cardiographic criteria for thrombolytic therapy, not many patients are eligible for this kind of reperfusion therapy. In contrast to the low sensitivity for myocardial infarction, ST elevation on ECG is associated with a specificity of 90 %. Only 10 % of new ECG changes in acute myocardial infarction are secondary to aortic dissection, coronary embolization, or vasospasm.

Serum Markers of Cardiac Damage

Myocardial necrosis is associated with diffusion of intracellular macromolecules (serum cardiac markers) into the cardiac interstitium and ultimately in the microvasculature. The temporal rise and fall of serially obtained serum values and the degree of enzyme elevation are both helpful to determine onset and size of myocardial infarction.

Creatine Kinase

In the past measurement of the enzyme creatine kinase (CK) was the most important factor to determine myocardial necrosis. Although serum CK has a high sensitivity for enzymatic detection of acute myocardial infarction, the specificity is low.

Troponin T and I

The cardiac-specific enzymes troponin T (TnT) and troponin I (TnI) are now considered the preferred biomarkers for diagnosing acute myocardial infarction. Troponin T and I are proteins and subunits of the troponin complex which regulates the calcium-mediated contractile process of striated muscle. The amino acid sequence of both troponin TnT and TnI is different in cardiac than in skeletal muscle. This permits the production of antibodies that are specific for the cardiac form of both proteins. TnT and TnI are not detected in the peripheral circulation under normal circumstances; however, both TnT and TnI may be elevated in patients with end-stage heart failure due to ischemic or nonischemic cardiomyopathy, underlining the fact that both enzymes correlate with myocardial damage regardless of cause.

The sensitivity of TnT and TnI for detection of acute myocardial infarction within the first 3 h of chest pain does not exceed 30 %. The sensitivity increases up to 42 % within the first 6 h and up to 97 % within the first 24 h, but it is very low at the time when a reliable cardiac marker for early diagnosis of acute myocardial infarction is most needed. Maximum serum concentrations occur 8–16 h after onset of myocardial damage. Elevations may persist up to 10 days for TnI and up to 14 days for TnT. This prolonged time course makes a late diagnosis of myocardial infarction possible and LDH isoenzyme analysis is no longer recommended. After successful recanalization of the infarct-related artery, a rapid release of TnT and TnI may be observed (so-called washout phenomenon) and may be an indicator of reperfusion.

Therapy

Most studies that have evaluated optimal treatment of myocardial infarction have been conducted in middle-aged men. Fortunately, over the past decade more women were included in clinical trials and gender-specific data are emerging. The following chapter focuses on our current knowledge of efficacy and side effects of treatment of myocardial infarction in women.

Revascularization

Thrombolytic therapy

Myocardial necrosis occurs 20 min after coronary occlusion and reaches its maximum after 6 h. Reperfusion of the infarct-related artery within this time frame is crucial for myocardial salvage. Two possible modalities of coronary reperfusion are available: (a) mechanically with coronary angioplasty (with or without stent implantation); or (b) medically with thrombolytic agents. Despite the fact that coronary reperfusion in STEMI is most efficacious within the first 6 h after onset of chest pain, either reperfusion strategy should be offered to all patients within 12 h of symptoms. Primary angioplasty is most meaningful if "door to balloon" does not exceed 90 min. In patients with NSTEMI thrombolytic therapy is not indicated.

Endogenous spontaneous fibrinolysis occurs in 20 % of patients with acute myocardial infarction. Reperfusion rates after intravenous administration of a fibrinolytic agent approaches 75 %, depending on pharmacokinetics of the agent, time of injection (with respect to the onset of chest pain), patient population, and adjunctive medical therapy. Complete reperfusion is present if thrombolysis in myocardial infarction (TIMI)-III flow can be established (TIMI III flow equals normal blood flow). Intracoronary injection of a thrombolytic agent is less effective than intravenous administration of the thrombolytic agent.

There are no known gender differences in pharmacokinetics and response to fibrinolytic therapy (Woodfield et al. 1997). Reperfusion rates are similar for both genders after adjustment for age and confounding factors (Table 5.2). The Global Utilization of Streptokinase and Tissue Plasminogen Activator for Occluded Coronary Arteries (GUSTO-I) trial (Weaver et al. 1996) reported a 90-min patency rate (TIMI III flow) of 39 % in women and of 38 % in men. The combined TIMI II and TIMI III patency rate was 69 and 66.5 %, respectively. These data were substantiated by the Thrombolysis and Angioplasty in Myocardial Infarction (TAMI) trial (Lincoff et al. 1993) with reperfusion rates of 74.3 % in women and 72.2 % in men.

Only "Gruppo Italiano per lo Studio della Streptochinasi nell'Infarto Miocardico" (GISSI-2) found a gender difference in diabetic patients: ST-segment elevations returned less often to baseline in women than in men suggesting less complete reperfusion in women.

Table 5.2. Gender-specific reperfusion rate with thrombolytic therapy

Study	Men (%)	Women (%)
GUSTO I	67	69
TAMI	72	74

❶ Menstruation, even at the time of active bleeding, does not cause any bleeding complications and thus is no contraindication for thrombolytic therapy; therefore, fibrinolytic agents should not be withheld in young menstruating women with acute myocardial infarction.

Primary Percutaneous Transluminal Coronary Angioplasty

According to the American Heart Association (AHA) and the American College of Cardiology (ACC) primary angioplasty is indicated in patients with contraindications for thrombolytic therapy and patients in cardiogenic shock.

One of the first large prospectively conducted multicenter trials that compared primary angioplasty with thrombolytic therapy (100 mg frontloaded t-PA) and performed a separate analysis of the gender-specific outcome was the Primary Angioplasty in Myocardial Infarction (PAMI-I) trial (Grines et al. 1993; Stone et al. 1995). Of the 395 patients, 27 % were women. In-hospital mortality was 3.3 times higher in women than in men, primarily due to a significant higher in-hospital mortality rate of women age 65 years or older treated with t-PA. There was no significant gender difference in the primary angioplasty group in all age groups; however, 22 % of women age 65 years or older who received thrombolytic therapy, but only 6 % treated with primary angioplasty, died at the time of hospitalization. In men and in women younger than 65 years there was no difference in in-hospital mortality between the percutaneous transluminal coronary angioplasty (PTCA) group and the thrombolysis group (Fig. 5.3).

Primary angioplasty not only reduced in-hospital mortality in women but also complications, including early reinfarction and the incidence of stroke. There were 7 patients with intracranial bleeding, all in women age 65 years or older treated with t-PA. A small disadvantage for women undergoing primary PTCA was the higher incidence of vascular groin complications (3.8 vs 1.2 %) and need for blood transfusion (19.5 vs 7.9 %).

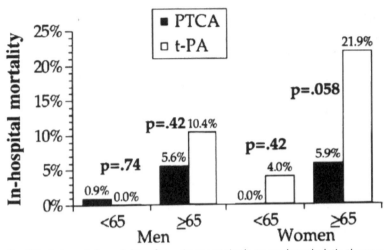

Fig. 5.3. In-hospital mortality after primary angioplasty or thrombolytic therapy. (From Stone et al. 1995)

Since the mid-1990s coronary stenting has become the mainstay of catheter-based interventions in both genders, even in patients with acute myocardial infarction; however, despite a dramatic in increase in stent usage limited information exists regarding the outcomes of women after stent implantation for acute myocardial infarction.

The Stent Primary Angioplasty in Myocardial Infarction Study Group trial included implantation of a Palmaz–Schatz stent. In this trial all patients slightly benefited from stent placement, but women less so than men. Women had a higher 6-month mortality and reinfarction rate, whereas late target revascularization rates were similar, but still slightly higher, than in men. In this study female gender was an independent predictor of the composite end points of death, reinfarction, and target vessel revascularization (TVR). Primary stenting improved the prognosis in men but not in women (Grines et al. 1999).

A recent small study from Italy, which examined gender differences in primary angioplasty or stenting (70 % of patients received stents) of patients with acute myocardial infarction, showed also a higher 6-month mortality rate for women (12 vs 7 %; $p=0.028$). Nonfatal reinfarction occurred in 3 % of the women and in 1 % of the men ($p=0.010$); however, in contrast to the previous study, the difference was no longer statistically significant after adjustment for baseline characteristics and age (Antoniucci et al. 2001).

Data from the Controlled Abciximab and Device Investigation to Lower Late Angioplasty Complications (CADILLAC) trial compared angioplasty with stenting, with or without Abciximab. The incidence of the primary composite end point of death, reinfarction, disabling stroke, and ischemia-driven TVR at 6 months was significantly lower in patients receiving coronary stents than in those undergoing balloon angioplasty. All patients significantly benefited from stenting; however – again – women did so less than men. The frequency of the composite end point was 15.2 % in women compared with only 8.8 % in men (Stone et al. 2002). Unfortunately, a subgroup analysis for women or in-depth evaluation of complications in women is not yet available.

⊘ Summary

In women primary angioplasty for acute myocardial infarction is more beneficial than thrombolytic therapy, particularly in women age 65 years or older and in women with diabetes and hypertension. Stenting in comparison with balloon angioplasty further improves prognosis, but less so in women than in men.

Since primary angioplasty is meaningful only if the door to balloon time (time from presentation in the emergency department until inflation of the balloon) does not exceed 2 h (ideally less than 90 min) and thus requires an experienced, well-staffed invasive angiography team on call 24 h a day, 7 days a week, it is very unlikely that primary angioplasty will be available for the majority of patients throughout the country; hence, primary angioplasty can be offered only to very few patients despite the fact that it is the therapy of choice in elderly women.

Thrombolysis Versus Primary PTCA

Factors that favor primary angioplasty are:
- Anterior myocardial infarction
- Inferior myocardial infarction with right ventricular involvement
- Age >75 years
- Cardiogenic shock
- Acute myocardial infarction associated with left heart failure or hemodynamic instability

Rescue PTCA after Thrombolysis of Acute Myocardial Infarction

When thrombolysis has failed to reperfuse the infarct vessel within 90 minutes (persistent ST-elevation on EKG and/or persistent chest pain) rescue PTCA is often performed. Data from the mid 1980's **however** demonstrated that routine PTCA in the first 24 hours after thrombolytic therapy is associated with a trend towards increased mortality (Michels and Yusuf 1995). In addition there is a higher risk of complications including reinfarction and need for emergency bypass surgery. The underlying pathophysiologic mechanism is most likely exacerbation of platelet activation and thrombosis at the site of plaque rupture due to mechanical injury. However, these studies did not specifically address the selective use of angiography and PTCA in the subset of patients with failed thrombolysis.

Only two randomized trials have specifically studied the use of rescue PTCA. Belenkie I et al. (1992) studied 28 patients with a persistently occluded infarct-related artery after thrombolytic therapy more than 3 hours after the onset of acute myocardial infarction; patients were randomly assigned to rescue PTCA ($n = 16$) or conservative treatment ($n = 12$). There was a nonsignificant trend for lower in-hospital mortality rates in the rescue PTCA group (6.3 % compared with 33.3 %; P = 0.13). The Randomized Evaluation of Salvage Angioplasty with Combined Utilization of Endpoints (RESCUE) study is the larger of the two trials that have specifically addressed rescue PTCA (Ellis 1994). The RESCUE study sample consisted of 151 patients with first anterior myocardial infarction who were treated with thrombolytic therapy and were shown to have an occluded infarctrelated artery (TIMI 0 or 1 flow) within 8 hours of pain onset. These patients were randomly assigned to undergo rescue PTCA ($n = 78$) or conservative medical management ($n = 73$). Recruitment of centers to participate in this trial was difficult because many investigators believed it would be unethical to withhold treatment in this setting. There was a trend towardss lower 30-day mortality (5.1 % compared with 9.6 %; $P = 0.18$) and less severe congestive heart failure (New York Heart Association functional class III or IV) (1.3 % compared with 7.0 %; $P = 0.11$) in the rescue PTCA group. A statistically significant benefit was reported in the rescue PTCA group for the combined outcome of death or severe congestive heart failure at 30 days (6.4 % compared with 16.6 %; $P = 0.05$).

Whether stenting and the use of glycoprotein IIb/IIIa receptor antagonists are able to further improve outcome after failed thrombolysis needs to be determined. Very little data and essentially no gender-specific data are

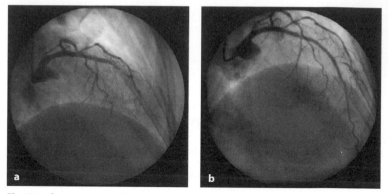

Fig. 5.4a, b. A 44-year-old premenopausal diabetic woman with complete occlusion of the LAD despite thrombolytic therapy with t-PA. She successfully underwent "rescue" coronary angioplasty with stent implantation

available yet. In addition, the question of whether a tailored approach with reduced dose lytics, GP IIb/IIIa receptor antagonists, and rescue PCI would be an alternative treatment strategy needs to be addressed as well. (An example of a rescue PTCA with implantation of a stent in a 58-year-old woman with acute anterior myocardial infarction is shown in Fig. 5.4.)

Medical Therapy of Acute Myocardial Infarction

Despite the fact that either pharmacological or mechanical reperfusion of the infarct-related artery is associated with the greatest reduction in mortality from acute myocardial infarction, adjunctive medical therapy is of the utmost importance as well. All patients with acute myocardial infarction should receive aspirin, a beta-blocker, and an antithrombin.

Since platelets play a pivotal role in the thrombotic response to rupture of a coronary artery plaque, platelet inhibition is critical. The agent most extensively studied has been aspirin and is recommended in all acute myocardial infarction patients.

The intravenous administration of beta-blockers reduces cardiac index, heart rate, and blood pressure. The net effect is reduction in myocardial oxygen consumption. Clinically, this translates into reduction of infarct size, recurrent ischemia, and reinfarction.

Despite continued controversy with respect to antithrombotic therapy, most investigators recommend an antithrombin as well given the major role played by thrombin in patients with acute myocardial infarction.

Aspirin

Only a few gender-specific data for treatment of acute myocardial infarction with aspirin are available. The Second International Study of Infarct Survival (ISIS-2) study was the largest trial of aspirin in acute myocardial infarction and showed a 23 % reduction in mortality from aspirin in both men and women; however only 25 % of the participating patients were women and a subgroup analysis for these women had inadequate statistical power.

A study from Israel, which examined aspirin in 2418 women with coronary artery disease, was associated with a reduction in all-cause mortality (RR 0.66; 95 % CI=0.47–0.93) and cardiovascular mortality (RR 0.61; 95 % CI=0.38–0.97) even after adjustment for age, risk factors, peripheral vascular disease, and previous infarction (Harpaz et al. 1996).

Within the first 24 h of acute myocardial infarction patients should receive 325 mg in chewable form. At least 81 mg daily are recommended for long-term treatment.

Beta-blockers

Three major studies (ISIS-1, the Timolol Myocardial Infarction Trial, and the Beta-Blocker Heart Attack Trial) suggest that reduction of cardiovascular mortality from beta-blockers is larger in women than in men. The Timolol Myocardial Infarction Trial reported a 41 % reduction in mortality for women, but of 35 % for men (Rodda 1983). The benefit is most pronounced in diabetics, however, independent of gender.

The AHA/ACC guidelines recommend metoprolol (i.v. in increments of 5 mg up to 15 mg/24 h) or atenolol (i.v. in increments of 10 mg up to 20 mg/24 h) at the time of presentation. Long-term therapy should include either metoprolol (50–100 mg/day) or atenolol (50–100 mg/day).

Unfractionated Heparin

Randomized trials conducted in the prethrombolytic era reported a reduction in the risk of stroke, reinfarction, and pulmonary embolism with intravenous unfractionated heparin in patients with acute myocardial infarction. There are conflicting data with respect to the risk–benefit ratio of heparin used as adjunct to aspirin and thrombolytic agents. For patients receiving either streptokinase or anistreplase there is no mortality benefit with intravenous administration of heparin. Since infarct-related artery patency rates are higher if heparin is given in patients treated with t-PA, heparin is indicated as adjunctive therapy to t-PA (and probable to tenecteplase and reteplase as well). Furthermore, heparin is commonly recommended in patients with large myocardial infarctions, anterior myocardial infarctions, patients in atrial fibrillation, and in patients with left ventricular thrombus. Recommended dosage is 60 units/kg as a bolus and 12 units/kg per hour. Target-activated partial thromboplastin time is 50–70 s.

Calcium Channel Blockers

Calcium channel blockers are not indicated. They do not reduce the risk of reinfarction or cardiovascular mortality. Two studies even suggest an increase in cardiovascular mortality (Held et al. 1989; Koenig et al. 1996).

ACE Inhibitors

Data from the Survival and Ventricular Enlargement (SAVE) trial (Pfeffer et al. 1992) revealed a smaller mortality rate reduction in cardiovascular mortality for women than in men (4 vs 28 %). The Trandolapril Cardiac Evaluation (TRACE) trial showed similar findings: women had a reduction in all-cause mortality of 10 %, but men of 26 %; however, a meta-analysis of several large-scale trials and data from 100,000 patients (ACE Inhibitor Myocardial Infarction Collaborative Group) did not find gender differences. Both men and women benefited from early administration of ACE inhibitor in the setting of an acute myocardial infarction, especially patients with ejection fractions less than 40 %.

However, theoretically a gender-specific response to ACE inhibitors is possible given the fact that there are gender differences in the renin-angiotensin system and serum levels of renin correlate inversely proportional with serum levels of estradiol (Schunkert et al. 1997). Future studies will elucidate these interesting interactions.

In essence, all patients with acute myocardial infarction should be treated with ACE inhibitors and in particular those with reduced left ventricular systolic function.

Nitrates

Despite the fact that nitrates are commonly used in the treatment of acute myocardial infarction, their impact on cardiovascular mortality remains unclear. A meta-analysis of six trials (Yusuf et al. 1988) found a reduction in cardiovascular mortality of 45 % if nitrates were given intravenously during the early phase of an acute myocardial infarction; however, these data did not reach statistical significance. Gender-specific data are not available at all.

Complications

Most studies report a higher incidence of complications in women with acute myocardial infarction than in men. (Fig. 5.5; Fiebach et al. 1990; Jenkins et al. 1994; Goldberg et al. 1993; Kannel et al. 1979; Malacrida et al. 1998; Weaver et al. 1996) Women are particularly at higher risk for:
- Cardiogenic shock
- Congestive heart failure
- Reinfarction
- Peripheral bleeding
- Stroke

Since most of these studies did not consistently adjust for age and comorbid conditions, the true degree of gender differences remains uncertain; however, data from the GUSTO trial showed a higher incidence of nonfatal complications even after adjustment for age. For example, in this trial the reinfarction rate for women was 5.1 % in contrast to 3.6 % for men. The Secondary Prevention Israeli Reinfarction Nifedipine Trial (SPRINT; Kornowski et al. 1995) demonstrated similar data and furthermore came to the conclusion that clinical predictors of reinfarction differ for men and women. Diabetes mellitus, congestive heart failure, cardiomegaly, and angina after myocardial infarction were clinical predictors of reinfarction in women but not in men. If peripheral vascular disease was present, women were twice as likely as men to suffer a reinfarction.

The most detrimental complication is stroke. Most strokes (hemorrhagic and nonhemorrhagic) occur in patients treated with thrombolytics. The GUSTO study found that women have a twofold higher risk of stroke independent of age or hypertension. The reasons for the greater risk of stroke remain to be determined. It had been speculated that this was due to overdose of the thrombolytic agent with regard to body size; however, after adjustment for weight in a series including more than 8000 patients, no association between body size and stroke could be seen. Pos-

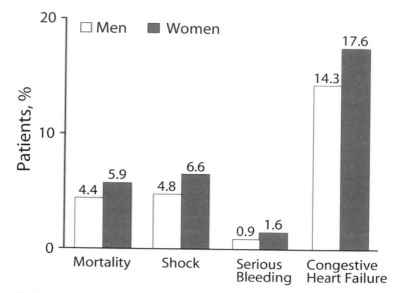

Fig. 5.5. Serious events after treatment with thrombolytic therapy and adjustment for age and differences in baseline characteristics (GUSTO I). (From Weaver et al. 1996)

sibly the higher incidence of hypertension in women with acute myocardial infarction may play an important role. In Primary Angioplasty in Myocardial Infarction (PAMI) trial 5.3 % of the women who underwent thrombolysis with t-PA suffered a cerebral bleeding, but only 0.7 % of the men. Overall hemorrhagic complications are more common in women treated with thrombolytic therapy than in men (Lincoff et al. 1993; White et al. 1993).

Prognosis

Assessment of mortality data for women with acute myocardial infarction is difficult for several reasons:
1. Most acute myocardial infarction studies up to the 1990s included only a relatively small number of women and even less women over the age of 75 years.

2. Study designs are not uniform and therefore studies are difficult to compare.
3. Entry criteria for studies are strict and therefore study patients may not be representative of actual myocardial infarction patients treated in the community. Furthermore, not only the time frame (in-hospital-, early-, or 30-day-, 6-month-, and 1-year mortality), but also kind of treatment (i.e., thrombolysis or not) and adjustment for age and confounding factors have to be taken into account.

Mortality in Acute Myocardial Infarction (With and Without Thrombolysis)

In 1995 Vaccarino et al. published an excellent review of gender differences in mortality after myocardial infarction and tried to understand the reported inconsistencies. Twenty-seven studies from 1966 until 1994 that controlled at least for age had 30 or more outcome events evaluated. Studies with and without thrombolytic therapy were included. Without adjustment for age the in-hospital and early mortality was 40 % higher in women than in men. With adjustment women had only a 20 % higher risk of dying that reached statistical significance in only two studies. Six of the 27 studies made adjustments for cardiovascular risk factors and comorbidities. All six trials found a relative risk (RR) greater than 1.0, but only three studies were statistically significant. Vaccarino et al. (1995) concluded that women do have a higher in-hospital and early mortality, but most (if not all) of the increased risk is due to the woman's older age at the time of presentation and the higher incidence of cardiovascular risk factors and comorbid conditions. A second analysis with respect to 1-year mortality demonstrated similar findings and there was even a trend for improved survival in women. It appears that women who survive the very early phase of acute myocardial infarction do even better than men.

However, younger women (<age 50 years) who have a myocardial infarction may represent a distinct group in terms of risk factors and pathophysiology. Data from the National Registry of Myocardial Infarction demonstrated that up to age 75 years all women had a higher overall mortality during hospitalization than men (16.7 % among women and 11.5 % among men), but that for women less than 50 years the mortality rate was even higher and more than twice that for men (Fig. 5.6). Differences in

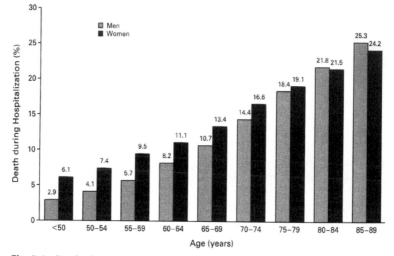

Fig. 5.6. Gender-based differences in early mortality after myocardial infarction. (From Vaccarino et al. 1999)

medical history, the clinical severity of the infarction, and early management (i.e., thrombolysis) accounted for only approximately one-third of the difference in the risk in the younger women.

The pathophysiology in premenopausal women may differ from the more common atherosclerotic disease of older women. It could be shown that female coronary artery lesions are more lipid filled, rich in macrophages, and less densely fibrous. They may be more prone to instability. This is in accordance with the fact that younger women have less narrowing of the coronary arteries than older women. In addition, a hypercoagulable state or spasm may be involved in the etiology of myocardial infarction in younger women as well.

Mortality in the Pre-thrombolytic Era (Mid-1960s to Early-1980s)

According to the Framingham Heart Study the 30-day mortality was significantly higher in women than in men (28 vs 16 %). A large multicenter trial from Israel reported an in-hospital mortality of 23 % in women and 16 % in men, even after adjustment for age and comorbid condition.

Mortality in the Thrombolytic Era (1980 to present)

Thrombolytic therapy has a substantial positive impact on mortality. All major placebo-controlled trials show an overall 17–45 % reduction in mortality in both men and women; however, gender-specific data are conflicting. Most of the major thrombolysis studies – ISIS-2, Anglo-Scandinavian Study of Early Thrombolysis (ASSET; Wilcox et al. 1988), GUSTO-I, and GISSI-I – demonstrated a twofold higher early mortality (up to 21–35 days) in women than in men (Table 5.3). The gender difference was especially striking in the first 7 days of the myocardial infarction (Fig. 5.7);

Table 5.3. Mortality after thrombolytic therapy without adjustment for age, risk factors, and angiographic findings

Study	Follow-up	Therapy	Mortality women (%)	Mortality men (%)
GISSI-1	3 weeks	SK	18.5	8.8
	1 year	SK	28.3	14.5
ISIS-2	5 weeks	SK	13.3	7.9
ASSET	4 weeks	rt-PA	8.6	6.8
GUSTO	4 weeks	SK	11.5	5.9
	4 weeks	rt-PA	10.2	5.0

SK streptokinase, *rt-PA* recombinant tissue plasminogen activator, *GISSI-1* Gruppo Italiano per lo Studio della Streptochinasi nell'Infarto Miocardio, *ISIS-2* Second International Study of Infarct Survival, *ASSET* Anglo-Scandinavian Study of Early Thrombolysis, *GUSTO* Global Utilization of Streptokinase and Tissue Plasminogen Activator for Occluded Coronary Arteries

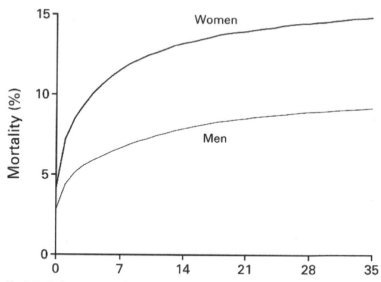

Fig. 5.7. Early outcome of acute myocardial infarction in women and men (ISIS 3). (From Malacrida 1999)

Table 5.4. Mortality after thrombolytic therapy with adjustment for age, risk factors, and angiographic findings

Study	Therapy	Follow-up	RR	p value
International t-PA/SK	SK, rt-PA	In-hospital	1.11	NS
	SK+rt-PA	6 months	1.02	NS
TAMI	UK, rt-PA, UK+rt-PA	In-hospital	1.31	NS
TIMI II	rt-PA	6 weeks	1.54	0.01
		1 year	1.39	NS

Relative risk (*RR*) comparison between women and men. *SK* streptokinase, *rt-PA* recombinant tissue plasminogen activator, *UK* urokinase, *NS* not significant, *International t-PA/SK* International Tissue Plasminogen Activator/Streptokinase Mortality Study, *TAMI* Thrombolysis and Angioplasty in Myocardial Infarction, *TIMI* Thrombolysis in Myocardial Infarction

however, in studies which made adjustments for age and confounding factors, this difference was essentially eliminated. In these studies gender differences did not reach statistical significance (Table 5.4). The GUSTO-I study reported conflicting data. Woodfield et al. (1997) found a 30-day mortality of 13 % in women and of 5 % in men. This gender difference persisted even after adjustment for age, diabetes mellitus, resting heart rate, and systolic blood pressure (RR=2.2). Another analysis of the same data did not find a gender difference with respect to 30-day mortality (RR=1.06; Moen et al. 1997).

◗ Summary

The following conclusions have been reached:

1. Women with acute myocardial infarction are older than men and have a higher incidence of cardiovascular risk factors.
2. Women present more often with NSTEMI than with STEMI.
3. Women have a higher incidence of complications with acute myocardial infarction than men do, in particular
   - Cardiogenic shock
   - Congestive heart failure
   - Reinfarction
   - Peripheral bleeding
   - Stroke
4. Despite similar rates of reperfusion with thrombolytic therapy, women have a higher risk of cerebral bleeding that can essentially be eliminated with primary angioplasty.
5. Women have a higher unadjusted early mortality after myocardial infarction than men. Despite the fact that after adjustment for age and cardiovascular risk factors the risk is only marginally elevated, gender remains an independent risk factor for mortality in acute myocardial infarction.

Influence of Gender on the Referral for Coronary Angiography in Patients with Acute Myocardial Infarction

Up to the mid-1990s less women than men underwent diagnostic cardiac catheterization in the setting of an acute myocardial infarction. It remains to be determined whether this was due to an "overuse" of coronary an-

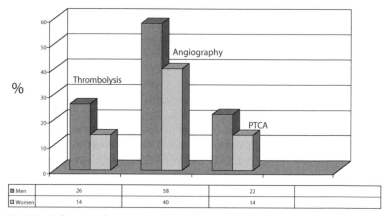

▣ Men	26	58	22
▢ Women	14	40	14

Fig. 5.8. Influence of gender on use of thrombolytic therapy and on referral to coronary angiography and percutaneous transluminal coronary angioplasty (*PTCA*). (From Maynard et al. 1992)

giography in men or a gender-based bias toward less frequent angiography in women. In most studies – the Myocardial Infarction Data Acquisitions System (MIDAS), Myocardial Infarction Triage and Intervention (MITI), and Sex Differences in the Management of Coronary Artery Disease/Survival and Ventricular Enlargement Investigators (SAVE) – gender still influenced referral patterns to coronary angiography even after adjustment for age and comorbid conditions (Fig. 5.8; Kostis et al. 1994; Maynard et al. 1992; Steingart et al. 1991). Only Funk and Griffey (1992) did not find a difference in the frequency of cardiac catheterization in men and women after adjustment for age and confounding factors. Recent evidence suggests that there is no difference in the usage of coronary angiography in the postinfarction period; however, further data have to be obtained.

References

ACE Inhibitor Myocardial Infarction Collaborative Group (1998) Indications for ACE inhibitors in the early treatment of acute myocardial infarction: systemic overview of individual data from 100,000 patients in randomized trials. Circulation 98(19):2202–2212

American Heart Association (1999) Heart and Stroken Statistical Update 1999. American Heart Association, Dallas/TX, vol 11

Antoniucci D, Valenti R, Moschi G et al. (2001) Sex-based differences in clinical and angiographic outcomes after primary angioplasty or stenting for acute myocardial infarction. Am J Cardiol 87:289–293

Becker RC, Terrin M, Ross R et al. (1994) Comparison of clinical outcomes for women and men after acute myocardial infarction. The Thrombolysis in Myocardial Infarction (TIMI-II) Investigators. Ann Intern Med 120:6345

Belenkie I, Traboulsi M, Hall CA et al. (1992) Rescue angioplasty during myocardial infarction has a beneficial effect on mortality: a tenable hypothesis. Can J Cardiol 8:357–362

Beta-Blocker Heart Trial Research Group (1982) A randomized trial of propranolol in patients with acute myocardial infarction. I. Mortality results. JAMA 247:1707–1714

De Jaegere PP, Arnold AA, Balk AH, Simoons ML (1992) Intracranial hemorrhage in association with thrombolytic therapy: incidence and clinical predictive factors. J Am Coll Cardiol 19:289–294

Demirovic J, Blackburn H, McGovern PG, Luepker R, Sprafka JM, Gilbertson D (1995) Sex differences in early mortality after acute myocardial infarction (the Minnesota Heart Survey). Am J Cardiol 75:1096–1101

Dittrich H, Gilpin E, Nicod P, Cali G, Henning H, Ross J jr (1988) Acute myocardial infarction in women: influence of gender on mortality and prognostic variables. Am J Cardiol 62:1–7

Ellis SG, Silva ER da, Heyndrickx G et al. (1994) Randomized comparison of rescue angioplasty with conservative management of patients with early failure of thrombolysis for acute anterior myocardial infarction. Circulation 90:2280–2284

Fiebach NH, Viscoli CM, Horwitz RI (1990) Differences between women and men in survival after myocardial infarction. Biology or methodology? JAMA 236:1092–1096

FRESCO-Trial: Antoniucci D, Santoro GM, Bolognese L et al. (1998) A clinical trial comparing primary stenting of the infarct-related artery with oprimal primary angioplasty for acute myocardial infarction. Results from the florence randomized elective stenting in acute coronary occlusions (Fresco) trial. J Am Coll Cardiol 31:496–501

Funk M, Griffey KA (1992) Relation of gender to the use of cardiac procedures in acute myocardial infarction. Am J Cardiol 74:1170–1173

Fuster V, Badimon L, Badimon JJ, Chesebro JH (1992) The pathogenesis of coronary artery disease and the acute coronary syndromes. N Engl J Med 326:310–318

Goldberg RJ, Gorak EJ, Yarzebski J et al. (1993) A community-wide perspective of sex differences and temporal trends in the incidence and survival rates after acute myocardial infarction and out-of-hospital deaths caused by coronary heart disease. Circulation 87:1947–1953

Greenland P, Reicher-Reiss H, Goldbourt U, Behar S (1991) In-hospital and 1-year-mortality in 1,524 women after myocardial infarction: comparison with 4,315 men. Circulation 83:484–491

Grines Cl, Browne KF, Marco J et al. (1993) A comparison of immediate angioplasty with thrombolytic therapy for acute myocardial infarction. The Primary Angioplasty in Myocardial Study Group. N Engl J Med 328:673–679

Grines CL, Cox DA, Stone GW et al. (1999) Coronary angioplasty with or without stent implantation for acute myocardial infarction. N Engl J Med 341:1949–1956

Gruppo Italiano per lo Studio della Streptochinasi nell'Infarto Miocardico (GISSI) (1986) Effectiveness of intravenous thrombolytic treatment in acute myocardial infarction. Lancet 1:397–401

Gurwitz JH, McLaughlin TJ, Willison DJ et al. (1997) Delayed hospital presentation in patients who have had acute myocardial infarction. Ann Intern Med 126:593–599

Harpaz D, Benderly M, Goldbourt U et al. (1996) Effect of aspirin on mortality in women with symptomatic or silent myocardial ischemia. Israeli BIP Study Group. Am J Cardiol 78:1215–1219

Held PH, Yusuf S, Furberg CD (1989) Calcium channel blockers in acute myocardial infarction and unstable angina: an overview. BMJ 299:1187–1192

Hochman JS, McCabe CH, Stone PH et al. (1997) Outcome and profile of women and men presenting with acute coronary syndromes: a report from TIMI IIIB. Thrombolysis in Myocardial Infarction (TIMI) Investigators. J Am Coll Cardiol 30:141–181

ISIS-1 Collaborative Group (1986) Randomized trial of intravenous atenolol among 16,027 cases of suspected acute myocardial infarction. Lancet 2:57–67

ISIS-2 (Second International Study of Infarct Survival) Collaborative Group (1988) Randomised trial of intravenous streptokinase, oral aspirin, both or neither among 17,187 cases of suspected acute myocardial infarction. ISIS-2. Lancet 2:349–260

ISIS-2 Collaborative Group (1987) Randomized factorial trial of high-dose intravenous streptokinase, of oral aspirin and of intravenous heparin in acute myocardial infarction. ISIS (International Studies of Infarct Survival) pilot study. Eur Heart J 8:634–642

Jenkins JS, Flaker GC, Nolte B et al. (1994) Causes of higher in-hospital mortality in women than in men after acute myocardial infarction. Am J Cardiol 73:319–322

Kannel WB, Abbott RD (1984) Incidence and prognosis of unrecognized myocardial infarction: an update on the Framingham study. N Engl J Med 311:1144–1147

Kannel WB, Sorlie P, McNamara PM (1979) Prognosis after initial myocardial infarction: the Framingham Study. Am J Cardiol 44:53–59

Karlson BW, Herlitz J, Hartford M (1994) Prognosis in myocardial infarction in relation to gender. Am Heart J 128:477–483

Koenig W, Lowel H, Lewis M, Hormann A (1996) Long-term survival after myocardial infarction: relationship with thrombolysis and discharge medication: results of the Augsburg Myocardial Infarction Follow-up Study 1985–1993. Eur Heat J. 17:1199–1206

Kornowski R, Goldbourt U, Boyko V, Behar S (1995) Clinical predictors of reinfarction among men and women after a first myocardial infarction. Secondary Prevention Israeli Reinfarction Nifedipine Trial (SPRINT) Study Group. Cardiology 86:163–168

Kostis JB, Wilson AC, O'Dowd K et al. (1994) Sex differences in the management and long-term outcome of acute myocardial infarction. A statewide study. MIDAS Study Group. Myocardial Infarction Data Acquisition system. Circulation 90:1715–1730

Libby P (1995) Molecular bases of the acute coronary syndromes. Circulation 91:2844–2850

Lincoff AM, Califf RM, Ellis SG et al. (1993) Thrombolytic therapy for women with myocardial infarction: is there a gender gap? Thrombolysis and Angioplasty in Myocardial Infarction (TAMI) Study Group. J Am Coll Cardiol 22:1780–1787

Maggioni AP, Franzosi MG, Santoro E et al. (1992) The risk of stroke inpatient with acute myocardial infarction after thrombolytic and antithrombotic treatment. Gruppo Italiano per lo Studio della Sopravvivenza nell'InfartoMiocardico II (GISSI-2) and the International Study Group. N Engl J Med 327:1–6

Malacrida R, Genoni M, Maggioni AP et al. (1998) A comparison of the early outcome of acute myocardial infarction in women and men. N Engl J Med 338:8–14

Marrugat J, Anto JM, Sala J, Masia R (1994) Influence of gender in acute and long-term cardiac mortality after a first myocardial infarction. REGICOR Investigators. J Clin Epidemiol 47:111–118

Maynard C, Litwin PE, Martin JS, Weaver WD (1992) Gender differences in the treatment and outcome of acute myocardial infarction: results from the Myocardial Infarction Triage and Intervention (MITI) Registry. Arch Intern Med 152:972–976

Meischke H, Eisenberg MS, Larsen MP (1993) Prehospital delay interval for patients who use emergency medical services: the effect of heart related medical conditions and demographic variables. Ann Emerg Med 22:1597–1601

Michels KB, Yusuf S (1995) Does PTCA in acute myocardial infarction affect mortality and reinfarction rates? A quantitative overview (meta-analysis) of the randomized clinical trials. Circulation 91:476–485

Moen EK, Asher CR, Miller DP et al. (1997) Long-term follow-up of gender-specific outcomes after thrombolytic therapy for acute myocardial infarction from the GUSTO-I Trial. J Womens Health 6:285–293

Murabito JM, Evans JC, Larson MG, Levy D (1993) Prognosis after the onset of coronary artery disease. An investigation of differences in outcome between the sexes according to initial coronary disease presentation. Circulation 88:2548–2555

Pfeffer MA, Braunwald E, Moye LA et al. (1992) Effect of captopril on mortality and morbidity in patients with left ventricular dysfunction after myocardial infarction: results of the Survival and Ventricular Enlargement Trail. The SAVE Investogators. N Engl J Med 327:669–677

Puletti M, Sunseri L, Curione M et al. (1984) Acute myocardial infarction: sex-related differences in prognosis. Am Heart J 108:63–66

Robinson K, Conroy RM, Mulcahy R, Hickey N (1988) Risk factors and in-hospital course of first episode of myocardial infarction or acute coronary insufficiency in women. J Am Coll Cardiol 11:932–936

Rodda BE (1983) The Timolol Myocardial Infarction Study: an evaluation of selected variables. Circulation 67:1101–1106

Savage MP, Krolewski AS, Kenien GG et al. (1988) Acute myocardial infarction in diabetes mellitus and significance of congestive heart failure as a prognostic factor. Am J Cardiol 62:665–669

Schmidt SB, Borsch MA (1990) The prehospital phase of acute myocardial infarction in the era of thrombolysis. Am J Cardiol 65:1411–1415

Schunkert H, Danser AH, Hense HW et al. (1997) Effects of estrogen replacement therapy on the renin-angiotensin system in post-menopausal women. Circulation 95:39–45

Smith JW, Marcus FI, Serokman R (1984) Prognosis of patient with diabetes mellitus after acute myocardial infarction. Am J Cardiol 54:718–721

Steingart RM, Packer M, Hamm P et al. (1991) Sex differences in the management of coronary artery disease. Survival and Ventricular Enlargement (SAVE) Investigators. N Engl J Med 325:226–230

Stone PH, Muller JE, Hartwell T et al. (1989) The effect of diabetes mellitus on prognosis and serial left ventricular function after acute myocardial infarction: contribution of both coronary disease and diastolic left ventricular dysfunction to the adverse prognosis. The MILIS Study Group. J Am Coll Cardiol 14:49–57

Stone Gw, Grines Cl, Browne KF et al. (1995) Comparison of in-hospital outcome in men versus women treated by either thrombolytic therapy or primary angioplasty for acute myocardial infarction. Am J Cardiol 75:987–992

Stone GW, Grines CL, Cox D et al. (2002) Comparison of angioplasty with stenting. With or without ABCIXIMAB, in acute myocardial infarction. N Engl J Med 346:957–966

Suryapranata H, van't Hof AWJ, Hoorntje JCA et al. (1998) Randomized comparison of coronary stenting with balloon angioplasty in selected patients with acute myocardial infarction. Circulation 97:2502–2505

Vaccarino V, Krumholz HM, Berkman LF, Horwitz RI (1995) Sex differences in mortality after myocardial infarction: is there evidence for an increased risk for women? Circulation 91:1861–1871

Vaccarino V, Parsons L, Every NR et al. (1999) for the National Registry of Myocardial Infarction 2 Participants. Sex-Based Differences in early Mortality after Myocardial Infarction. N Engl J Med 341:217–225

Weaver WD, White HD, Wilcox RG et al. (1996) Comparisons of characteristics and outcomes among women and men with acute myocardial infarction treated with thrombolytic therapy. GUSTO-I Investigators. JAMA 275:777–782

White HD, Barbash GI, Modan M et al. (1993) After correcting the worse baseline characteristics, women treated with thrombolytic therapy for acute myocardial infarction have the same mortality and morbidity as men except for a higher incidence of hemorrhagic stroke. The Investigators of the International Tissue Plasminogen Activator/Streptokinase Mortality Study. Circulation. 1993;88:2097–103

Wilcox RG, von der Lippe G, Olsson CG et al. (1988) Trial of tissue plasminogen activator for mortality reduction in acute myocardial infarction. Anglo-Scandinavian Study of Early Thrombolysis (ASSET). Lancet 2:525–530

Wilkinson P, Laji K, Ranjadayalan K, parsons L, Timmis AD (1994) Acute myocardial infarction in women: survival analysis in first six months. Br Med J 309:566–569

Woodfield SL, Lundergan CF, Reiner JS et al. (1997) Gender and acute myocardial infarction: is there a different response to thrombolysis? J Am Coll Cardiol 29:35–42

Zuanetti G, Latini R, Maggioni AP et al. (1993) Influence of diabetes on mortality in acute myocardial infarction: data from the GISSI-2 study. J Am Coll Cardiol 22:1788–1794

Acute Coronary Syndromes

Non-ST-Elevation Myocardial Infarction/
Unstable Angina 116

Definition 118

Presentation 118

Diagnosis 119

Therapy 120

References 131

Non-ST-Elevation Myocardial Infarction/Unstable Angina

The spectrum of acute coronary syndromes reaches from acute myocardial ischemia without ECG changes and without enzyme rise to non-ST-elevation myocardial infarction (NSTEMI; previously non-Q-wave myocardial infarction) with subsequent development of Q-waves on the ECG despite initial classification as non-Q-wave myocardial infarction (2–15 % of patients with NSTEMI). Women present more often with NSTEMI (25 %) than men (16 %). The finding that women have a higher tendency for platelet aggregation than men correlates well with the finding that thrombi associated with NSTEMI are rich in platelets, whereas thrombi associated with STEMI are rich in erythrocytes and fibrin. This gender difference plays an important role in treatment of acute coronary syndromes.

Patients with acute coronary syndromes have a high risk of in-hospital mortality. In patients with angina refractory to medical therapy (defined as angina lasting longer than 10 min despite aspirin, nitroglycerin, beta-blocker, and heparin) it reaches 20 %. In contrast, the average in-hospital mortality rate for patients with STEMI and thrombolytic therapy is 6 %.

Factors that increase or decrease the likelihood that chest pain is due to coronary artery disease (CAD) do not differ for men and women. Most helpful in establishing or rejecting the diagnosis is the character of symptoms and ECG changes (Table 6.1); however, it should be kept in mind that women are, on average, 10 years older than men at the time of presentation and that a higher percentage of women than men present with atypical symptoms.

Table 6.1. Likelihood of significant coronary artery disease (CAD) in patients presenting with symptoms suggestive of acute coronary syndrome

High	Intermediate	Low
History of CAD		

Typical angina
  Man   >60 years
  Woman >70 years
	Typical angina
	  Man <60 years
	  Woman <70 years
		Nonspecific chest pain

ECG changes with pain		One risk factor (not diabetes)
ST depression >1 mm		

	Probable angina
	  Man >60 years
	  Woman >70 years
		T-wave flattening
		
		Normal ECG

Symmetric T-wave inversions in several precordial leads	Atypical angina with diabetes or with more than two risk factors (diabetes excluded)	
	ST depression of 0.05–1 mm T-wave inversion with prominent R	

A "high probability" refers to a likelihood of CAD >85 %. "Intermediate probability" ranges between 15 and 85 % and a "low probability" is a likelihood <15 %.

Definition

The diagnosis of an acute coronary syndrome can be made if one of the following is present:
- Angina at rest (>20 min), and/or
- Exertional angina less than 2 months duration and Canadian Cardiovascular Society (CCS) class III or IV, or
- Progression of angina CCS class I or II to CCS class III or IV over the previous days or weeks

Presentation

Acute coronary syndromes present with a large variety of symptoms. On one side of the spectrum there is a woman with new onset of exertional angina for the previous 2 months, and on the other side a patient with severe angina at rest with radiation of her pain into the arm and neck and associated with nausea and diaphoresis. Due to the heterogeneity of the disease and the high frequency of atypical symptoms in women, early diagnosis of CAD/unstable angina in the female population is difficult. Furthermore, both factors are frequently the reason that the diagnosis is made too late or not at all; on the other hand, due to the fact that women have a higher incidence of rest angina than men, many women are falsely classified as patients with an "acute coronary syndrome" but who retrospectively do not have coronary heart disease.

 Atypical symptoms in women very suggestive of unstable angina are new onset of shortness of breath or indigestion, in particular in postmenopausal and/or elderly women with multiple risk factors.

For prognostic reasons and guidance in subsequent therapy it is meaningful to classify patients (independent of gender) with acute coronary syndromes into different risk groups (Table 6.2):
1. Patients at low risk
2. Patients at medium risk
3. Patients at high risk

Table 6.2. Clinical indicators of high, intermediate, and low risk in patients with acute coronary syndrome. *CAD* coronary artery disease. (Modified from Braunwald et al. 1994)

High risk	Intermediate risk	Low risk
Persistent pain >20 min	Angina at rest >20 min, pain free at presentation, but high or intermediate likelihood of CAD	Increasing frequency, duration, or intensity of angina
Pulmonary edema	Angina at rest >20 min, relieved with rest or nitroglycerin	Angina lower in threshold than in the past
Angina associated with new or worsening mitral regurgitation	New onset angina CCS class III or IV and high or intermediate likelihood of CAD	New onset angina (2 weeks to 2 months)
Angina with a S3 or left heart failure	Pathologic Q-waves or ST ST depression >1 mm in at least two consecutive leads	ECG normal or unchanged
Angina associated with hypotension	Age >65 years	

Diagnosis

Five percent of all patients with unstable angina have a normal ECG. The most common ECG changes seen with acute coronary syndromes are nonspecific ST-T-wave changes. Deep symmetrical T-waves in V1—V4 are very suggestive of ischemia in the left anterior descending artery distribution. Transient ST elevations are due to vasospasm, either in a normal coronary artery or on top of a pre-existing coronary artery stenosis. Dynamic ST-T-wave changes >1 mm are generally associated with high risk.

In all patients with high likelihood of coronary heart disease but with a normal initial ECG, serial ECGs should be obtained (every 30–60 min, at least three ECGs). Additionally, every change in clinical status (i.e., new pulmonary edema) or recurrent chest pain is a reason to obtain a repeat ECG.

Acute coronary syndromes with elevation of troponin I or T are classified as NSTEMI. It must be kept in mind that there is only a very fine line between definition of a NSTEMI and of "unstable angina" given the fact that many NSTEMIs are only associated with a very small enzyme leak (i.e., troponin of 7 ng/dl). At the time when troponin I or T measurements were not readily available these patients were felt to be only "unstable angina" patients.

Therapy

Although the pathophysiology of acute coronary syndromes is similar to that of an STEMI, it is not the same and therefore requires a different therapeutic approach. Both NSTEMI and STEMI are caused by rupture of an atherosclerotic plaque with subsequent platelet adhesion and aggregation and thrombus formation. The culprit coronary artery is occluded in 100 % of all STEMIs, however, only in 60 % of all NSTEMI cases. Additionally, as pointed out previously, thrombi associated with NSTEMI are rich in platelets, whereas STEMI is associated with thrombi rich in erythrocytes and fibrin. Based on this pathophysiology, it is understandable that thrombolytic therapy is ineffective in patients with NSTEMI and even may be detrimental due to the fact that thrombolytics "liberate" thrombin and hence may increase thrombus formation. In patients with acute coronary syndrome/NSTEMI inactivation of platelets is one of the most important steps in therapy.

Medical Therapy

According to the AHA/ACC guidelines all patients with an acute coronary syndrome should be treated with a thrombin inhibitor (heparin or hirudin) and with aspirin.

Aspirin

If the patient was not taking aspirin on a regular basis, the initial dose of aspirin (324 mg) should be given in chewable form.

Aspirin inhibits the enzyme cyclooxygenase and thus thromboxane-A2-dependent platelet aggregation. Aspirin has no effect on other factors that induce platelet aggregation, such as thrombin (thrombin is the most potent stimulus for platelet aggregation). Despite these limitations, aspirin has been shown to reduce the risk of myocardial infarction including re-infarction and cardiovascular mortality in all patients with acute coronary syndromes, women included (Cairns et al. 1985; Theroux et al. 1988). Gender-specific subgroup analyses are not yet available.

Unfractionated Heparin

Conflicting data exist with respect to treatment of acute coronary syndromes with unfractionated heparin. It still remains unclear whether the combination of unfractionated heparin with aspirin is of incremental benefit than either agent alone. A meta-analysis of the most important and largest trials found that the combination of aspirin with heparin reduces the combined end point of myocardial infarction and cardiovascular mortality by 56 % (decrease from 3.3 to 1.8 %; RR=0.44). Another study found that heparin alone is more beneficial than combination therapy. Optimal dosage and duration of heparin administration are still matter of debate as well. Most likely an infusion of less than 48 h has no effect on the incidence of myocardial infarction or mortality. If, however, 6–7 days of treatment are necessary remains to be determined. Subcutaneous administration is of little value. Gender-specific data are not available, either.

Low-Molecular-Weight Heparin

The use of low-molecular-weight heparin has become the standard of care in the management of patients with acute coronary syndromes.

Low-molecular-weight heparin has several advantages in comparison with unfractionated heparin:
- Direct thrombin inhibition
- A reliable anticoagulant effect due to little fluctuations in serum levels
- Fewer side effects: lesser risk of osteoporosis and thrombocytopenia

Over the past couple of years four major trials compared low-molecular-weight heparin with unfractionated heparin in patients with acute coronary syndromes. These trials examined efficacy and the risk of bleeding (Table 6.3). Gurfinkel et al (1995; therapy with nadroparin-calcium) found a reduction in in-hospital mortality from 5.7 to 0.0 %. The FRISC trial (therapy with dalteparin) reported a reduction in the combined end

Table 6.3. Low-molecular-weight heparin (LMWH) in comparison with unfractionated heparin (UH) in patients with acute coronary syndrome

Study	Follow-up	Death/myocardial infarction ASA + LMWH (%)	ASA + Standard
ESSENCE	30 days	6.2	7.7
Gurfinkel	In hospital	0.0	5.7
FRIC	6 days	3.9	3.6
FRISC	6 days	1.8	4.8

ASA aspirin, *Standard* unfractionated heparin, *ESSENCE* Enoxaparin in Unstable Angina and Non-Q-Wave Myocardial Infarction, *FRIC* Low Molecular Weight Heparin (Fragmin) in the Treatment of Unstable Coronary Artery Disease, *FRISC* Fragmin During Instability in Coronary Artery Disease

point of myocardial infarction and 6-day mortality from 4.8 to 1.8 %; however, long-term results (after 150 days) did not differ between the two treatment groups. In the ESSENCE trial (therapy with enoxaparin) myocardial infarction and cardiovascular mortality were reduced from 7.7 to 6.2 %. The FRIC trial only (therapy with fragmin) did not find any difference in outcome (3.6 % for low-molecular-weight heparin vs 3.9 % for unfractionated heparin). Major bleeding complications were similar for both forms of heparin. The FRISC trial reported that women given dalteparin (weight adjusted) had a higher incidence of minor bleeding complications compared with men, suggesting that a lower dose per kilogram of body weight may have the same efficacy in women but a better safety profile.

Given these data, low-molecular-weight heparin is indicated in all women with acute coronary syndrome at high or moderate risk for coronary events. It is more efficacious than unfractionated heparin, easier to use, and in addition, it does not require frequent measurements of PTT.

Unfortunately, gender-specific data are also not yet available.

Glycoprotein IIb/IIIa Receptor Antagonists

After plaque rupture and adhesion of platelets to the plaque, the glycoprotein (GP) IIb/IIIa receptor changes its configuration in such a way that binding of fibrinogen takes place which in turn causes platelet aggregation and eventually thrombus formation; thus, the GP IIb/IIIa receptor plays a crucial role in platelet aggregation and in the pathophysiology of acute coronary syndromes.

Three major commercially available GP IIb/IIIa receptor antagonists are in use:

1. Abciximab (previous name 7E3-Fab; a monoclonal antibody)
2. Eptifibatide (a peptide)
3. Tirofiban (a non-peptide; Table 6.4)

Eptifibatide (Integrelin) and tirofiban (Aggrastat) are classified as small molecules.

All agents have to be injected and do not show efficacy with oral administration. Lamifiban has been withdrawn from the market since its efficacy was too low.

Table 6.5 shows differences in pharmacokinetics, immunogenicity, and bleeding risk.

Five landmark trials (35 % of the participants were women, four of the trials are known as the "4P trials": PURSUIT, PRISM, PRISM-PLUS, PARAGON) established the now proven medical therapy of acute coronary syndromes with GP receptor antagonists.

Platelet GP-IIb/IIIa in Unstable Angina: Receptor Suppression Using Integrelin Therapy (PURSUIT) enrolled 10,948 patients with unstable angina or a NSTEMI. Within 24 h patients were randomized to either eptifibatide or placebo on top of their conventional medical therapy. After 30 days, there was a 1.5 % absolute and a 9.5 % relative reduction in the

Table 6.4. Classification of glycoprotein (GP) IIb/IIIa receptor antagonists

Form	GP IIb/IIIa receptor antagonist
Monoclonal antibody	Abciximab
Synthetic GP IIb/IIIa antagonists	
Peptide	Eptifibatide
Non-peptide	Tirofiban
	Lamifiban
Natural GP IIb/IIIa antagonist	Snake venom

Table 6.5. Pharmacological differences between the synthetic GP IIb/IIIa receptor antagonists and abciximab

	Abciximab	Eptifibatide, tirofiban
Binding to receptor	Irreversible	Reversible
Specificity	Low	High
Half-life	Long (4–6 h)	Short (30–120 min)
Duration of action	2–3 days	~4 h
Bleeding risk	High	Low
Immunogenicity	High	Absent

combined end-point myocardial infarction and/or death from coronary cause in the eptifibatide group with high bolus (180 µg/kg). Benefit was seen for almost all subgroups; however, women did not show a reduction in myocardial infarction or cardiac mortality with the exception for women in the United States (Fig. 6.1). The reasons remain unclear. Biological differences most likely are not the cause for the difference in outcome, since it could be shown that the degree of platelet inhibition by eptifibatide was similar for men and women. Since other trials with eptifibatide did not show any gender difference, the possible underlying cause may be differences in demographic variables and differences in the concomitant therapy.

The Platelet Receptor Inhibition in Ischemic Syndrome Management (PRISM) trial randomized 3000 patients with unstable angina or NSTEMI (32 % of whom were women) to tirofiban or heparin. Women treated with the GP-IIb/IIIa receptor antagonist had more benefit than men (Fig. 6.2). Given the fact that NSTEMIs are more common in women than in men and the fact that thrombi associated with NSTEMI are rich in platelets, it is understandable that treatment with GP-IIb/IIIa receptor antagonists is more efficacious in women than in men. In all patients there was a 36 % reduction in the common end point of "death, myocardial infarction, or refractory angina" after 48 h of treatment (5.9 % in the heparin group, 3.8 % in the tirofiban group). A reduced cardiovascular mortality was still seen after 30 days.

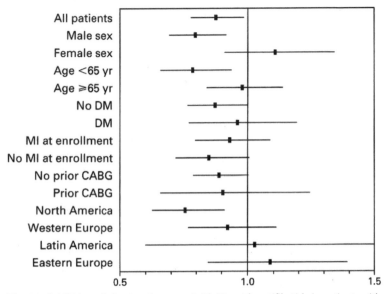

Fig. 6.1. Inhibition of platelet glycoprotein IIb/IIIa with eptifibatide in patients with acute coronary syndromes. (From PURSUIT Investigators 1998)

The Platelet Receptor Inhibition in Ischemic Syndrome Management in Patients Limited by Unstable Signs and Symptoms (PRISM-PLUS) trial was similar in design than the PRISM trial but enrolled high-risk patients only. Thirty percent of these patients had a history of percutaneous transluminal coronary angioplasty (PTCA) or coronary artery bypass grafting (CABG). Thirty-three percent of the 2000 participants were women. Patients were randomized to tirofiban alone, tirofiban plus heparin, and heparin alone. The "tirofiban alone"-group was prematurely discontinued because of a high 7-day mortality and myocardial infarction rate. After 30 days, the combination of tirofiban with heparin showed a 23 % reduction of cardiovascular events (18.5 vs 22.3 %) for both men and women. In men the incidence of cardiovascular events was reduced from 19 % (heparin) to 13.4 % for (heparin plus tirofiban). In women there was a reduction from 17.4 to 12.7 %, respectively. The benefit persisted for the following 6 months (27.7 vs 32.1 %). There was no difference in bleeding complications for the "heparin alone" or combination therapy.

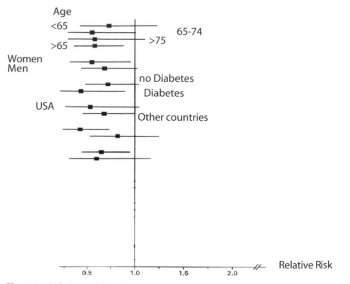

Fig. 6.2. Relative risk for the combined end point death, nonfatal myocardial infarction, or refractory ischemia in the PRISM trial. (From PRISM Investigators 1998)

The Platelet-IIa/IIIb Antagonist for the Reduction of Acute Coronary Syndrome Events in a Global Organization Network (PARAGON) trial randomized 2282 patients with unstable angina to lamifiban plus heparin or heparin alone. After 30 days, there was no difference in outcome between the treatment groups. Lamifiban is not used in clinical practice.

The Global Use of Strategies to Open Occluded Coronary Arteries (GUSTO) IV-ACS trial randomized 7800 patients with acute coronary syndromes and positive troponin or ECG changes to abciximab or placebo. Unexpectedly, there was no difference in outcome between either group.

The U.S. Food and Drug Administration recommends Integrelin or tirofiban in all patients with acute coronary syndromes who remain symptomatic after 1 h of conventional treatment and/or in all high-risk patients (see Table 6.2). It could be shown that patients with positive troponin have the highest benefit. Optimal dosages and duration of treatment are still a matter of investigation. Abciximab is not recommended for medical treatment of patients with acute coronary syndromes or

NSTEMI. It can be administered in patients prior to coronary intervention.

Besides therapy with platelet inhibitors and an anti-thrombin, treatment with beta-blocker and nitrates is recommended. Calcium channel blockers should be used with caution and only when beta-blockers are contraindicated. Unfortunately, gender-specific data with respect to medical treatment are not yet available; therefore, ways of treatment have to be based on studies in men.

Nitrates

As of yet, no randomized trial could demonstrate a reduction in cardiovascular mortality or rate of myocardial infarction with the use of nitrates for acute coronary syndromes. They are indicated for symptomatic relief of angina.

Beta-blockers

Beta-blockers are the cornerstone therapy for acute coronary syndromes. They not only reduce ischemic episodes and the risk of myocardial infarction, but also cardiovascular mortality in postinfarction patients.

Gender differences in pharmacology have been noted, but data from large randomized trials are not available.

Calcium Channel Blockers

In some studies calcium channel blockers were associated with an increase in mortality. Most data suggest that calcium channel blockers do not reduce the risk of recurrent myocardial infarction.

Verapamil or diltiazem can be used in patients with recurrent ischemia and/or in patients with atrial fibrillation and rapid ventricular response in whom beta-blockers are contraindicated.

Interventional Therapy

Diagnostic cardiac catheterization is crucial to determine the number and location of coronary artery stenoses and lesion morphology (i.e., whether an intracoronary thrombus is present or not). These findings not only allow a more detailed risk stratification, but are also the basis for further treatment (i.e., PTCA with or without stent implantation or CABG). Approximately, 10 % of all patients with acute coronary syndromes have no obstructive CAD, even those with ECG changes; however, in 6 % of patients symptoms are due to a left main stenosis.

All high-risk patients should undergo a diagnostic cardiac catheterization as soon as possible, and particularly patients with recurrent ischemia (demonstrated by either ongoing pain or recurrent ECG changes).

Besides "refractory ischemia," the ACC/AHA guidelines recommend a cardiac catheterization within the first 48 h after hospitalization for all patients with the following findings:

- Malignant arrhythmias
- Hypotension
- Heart failure and/or ejection fraction <40 %
- New or worsening mitral regurgitation
- Ventricle septal defect (VSD)
- Hemodynamic instability including cardiogenic shock

Patients with a history of PTCA with or without stent implantation, atherectomy, or CABG should undergo an invasive strategy as well. Given the fact that these recommendations were written before the use of GP-IIa/IIIb receptor antagonists and frequent use of stents, it is questionable whether medical treatment only is justified in all other patients. Four large randomized trials tried to answer this question and randomized all patients with acute coronary syndromes to either an early invasive or to a non-invasive strategy: the Thrombolysis in Myocardial Infarction (TIMI) IIIb trial (Anonymous), the Veterans Affairs Non Q Wave Infarction Strategies in Hospital (VANQWISH) trial (Boden et al. 1998), the Fast Revascularisation During In Stability in Coronary Artery Disease (FRISC) II trial (Anonymous), and the Treat Angina with Aggrastat and Determine Cost of Therapy with an Invasive or Conservative Strategy (TACTICS)TIMI 18 trial (Cannon et al. 1998). The TIMI IIIb and VANQWISH trials were conducted before introduction of GP-IIb/IIIa antagonists and stents. In FRISC II some of the patients received stents but no GP-IIb/IIIa antagonist. The TACTICS trial was the only trial that used both, stents and GP-IIa/IIIb antagonists. Forty-eight percent of patients in TIMI IIIb were women, but only 3 % of patients in VANQWISH; however, a subgroup analysis for women is not available for either of the four trials.

In TIMI IIIb and in VANQWISH the common end point of "cardiovascular mortality and reinfarction" did not differ between the invasive or conservative treatment groups; however, the need for repeat hospitalization, the length of stay, and the use of antianginal medication was less in the invasive group than in the conservative group. Furthermore, 64 % of patients with an initial conservative strategy required a revascularization procedure later.

In FRISC II the invasive strategy was superior to the conservative strategy: 9.4 % of patients of the invasive group, but 12.1 % of the conservative group, suffered either a nonfatal myocardial infarction or died from coronary cause within the first 6 months. Repeat hospitalization and angina was reduced by 50 % with the invasive strategy. Most striking were the differences in the high-risk population.

In TACTICS the invasive strategy was associated with further reduction in the common end point of "death, myocardial infarction, and repeat hospitalization": 7.4 vs 10.5 % after 30 days and 15.9 vs 19.4 % after 6 months. Patients in the high-risk category had the greatest benefit: There was a reduction from 30.6 to 19.5 % with an early invasive strategy. Women with low risk showed no significant benefit. The improved prognosis with an invasive strategy can most likely be attributed to the improved antiplatelet therapy due to GP-IIa/IIIb receptor antagonists and the use of stents.

Boersma et al. (1999) showed as well that early coronary intervention on top of medical treatment with GP-IIa/IIIb antagonists in patients with NSTEMI further reduces the cumulative incidence of cardiac death and nonfatal myocardial infarction than medical therapy alone (Fig. 6.3). Given these findings early cardiac catheterization, and if needed, early coronary intervention is the treatment of choice for all patients with acute coronary syndromes and elevated troponin.

As already mentioned, women not only are treated less aggressively than men, but are also less often referred for cardiac catheterization. Given the fact that at the time of presentation women more often than men belong to the high-risk category due to their older age and higher prevalence of diabetes mellitus and hypertension, women would benefit even more from an early invasive strategy. In order to substantially reduce cardiovascular mortality in women, the medical community has to change treatment habits from a more conservative to a more aggressive approach (see Fig. 6.4 for an example of an early intervention in a woman with NSTEMI).

◆ Summary

Acute coronary syndromes comprise unstable angina and non-ST-elevation myocardial infarction. Women frequently show atypical symptoms; however, factors that increase or decrease the likelihood that chest pain is

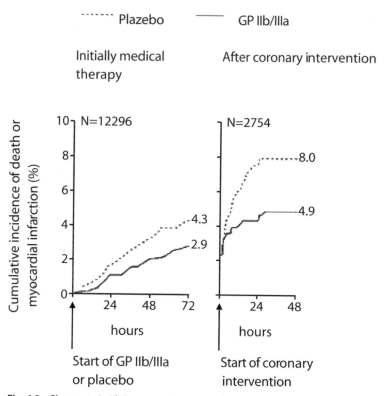

Fig. 6.3. Glycoprotein IIb/IIIa receptor antagonists in patients with acute coronary syndromes. (From Boersma et al. 1999)

due to CAD do not differ for men and women. Diagnostic tools are the same for men and women. Response to medical treatment and side effects may differ between genders, but future pharmacological research results have to be obtained. Women appear to benefit slightly more from glycoprotein IIb/IIIa antagonists than men. An early invasive strategy with early diagnostic cardiac catheterization and, if needed, with early revascularization (either PTCA with or without stent or CABG) reduces cardiovascular mortality even further in women at intermediate and at high risk.

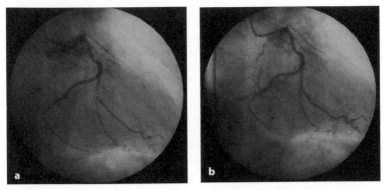

Fig. 6.4a, b. A 55-year-old woman with acute coronary syndrome. Her coronary angiogram revealed a high-grade stenosis with thrombus in the mid-circumflex that was successfully treated with angioplasty and stent implantation

References

Anonymous (1994) Invasive compared with non-invasive treatment in unstable coronary-artery disease: FRISC II prospective randomised multicentre study. Fragmin and Fast Revascularisation during InStability in Coronary artery disease Investigators. Lancet 354(9180):708–715

Ambrose JA, Dangas G (2000) Unstable angina: Current concepts of pathogenesis and treatment. Arch Int Med 160:25–37

Antman EM, McCabe CH, Gurfinkel EP et al. (1999) Enoxaparin prevents death and cardiac ischemic events in unstable angina/non-Q-wave myocardial infarction. Circulation 100:1593–1601

Bhatt DL, Topol EJ (2000) Current Role of Glycoprotein IIb/IIIa Inhibitors in Acute Coronary Syndromes. JAMA 284(12):1549–1558

Boden WE, O'Rourke RA, Crawford MH et al. (1998) Outcomes in patients with acute non-Q-wave myocardial infarction randomly assigned to aninvasive as compared with a conservative management strategy. Veterans Affairs Non-Q-Wave Infarction Strategies in Hospital (VANQWISH) Trial Investigators. N Engl J Med 338(25):1785–1792

Boersma E, Akkerhuis KM, Theroux P et al. (1999) Platelet glycoprotein IIb/IIa receptor inhibition in non-ST-elevation acute coronary syndromes:early benefit during medical treatment only, with additional protection during percutaneous coronary intervention. Circulation 100:2045–2048]

Braunwald E, Jones RH, Mark DB et al. (1994) Diagnosing and managing unstable angina. Circulation 90:613–622

Cairns JA, Gent M, Singer J et al. (1985) Aspirin, sulfinpyrazone, or both in unstable angina: results of a Canadian multicenter trial. N Engl. J Med. 313:1369–1375

Califf R (1999) Glycoprotein IIb/IIIa blockade and thrombolytics: Early lessons from the Speed and GUSTO IV trials. Am Heart J 138(1, Part 2):S12–S15

Cannon CP, Weintraub WS, Demopoulos LA et al. (1998) Invasive vs. conservative strategies in unstable angina and non-Q-wave myocardial infarction following treatment with tirofiban: rationale and study design of the international TAC-TICS-TIMI 18 Trial. Treat Angina with Aggrastat and determine Cost of Therapy with an Invasive or Conservative Strategy. Thrombolysis in Myocardial Infarction. Am J of Cardiol 82(6):731–736

Fragmin during Instability in Coronary Artery Disease (Frisc) Study Group (1996) Low-molecular-weight-heparin during instability in coronary artery disease. Lancet 347:561–568

Gurfinkel EP, Manos EJ, Mejail RI et al. (1995) Low molecular weight heparin vs. regular heparin or aspirin in the treatment of unstable angina and silent ischemia. J Am Coll Cardiol 2: 313–318

Klein W, Buchwald A, Hillis WS et al. (1997) Fragmin in unstable angina pectoris or in non-Q-wave acute myocardial infarction (the FRIC study). Fragmin in Unstable Coronary Artery Disease. Am J Cardiol 80(5A):30E–34E

Libby P (1995) Molecular bases of the acute coronary syndromes. Circulation 91:2844–2850

Neri Serneri GG, Modesti PA, Gensini GF et al. (1995) Randomised comparison of subcutaneous heparin, intravenous heparin, and aspirin in unstable angina. Lancet 345:1201–1204

Stone PH, Thompson B, Anderson HV et al. (1996) Influence of race, sex, and age on management of unstable angina and non-Q-wave myocardial infarction. The TI-MI III registry. JAMA 275:1104–1112

The PARAGON Investigators (1998) International, randomized, controlled trial of lamifiban (a platelet glycoprotein IIb/IIIa inhibitor), heparin, or both in unstable angina. Circulation 97:2386–2395

The PRISM Investigators (1998) A comparison of aspirin plus tirofiban with aspirin plus heparin for unstable angina. N Engl J Med 338: 1498–1505

The PRISM-PLUS Investigators (1998) Inhibition of the platelet glycoprotein IIb/IIIa receptor with tirofiban in unstable angina and non-Q-wave mocardial infarction. N Engl J Med 338:1488–1497

The PURSUIT Investigators (1998) Inhibition of platelet glycoprotein IIb/IIIa with eptifibatide in patients with acute coronary syndromes. N Engl J Med 339:436–443

Theroux P, Ouimet H, McCans J et al. (1988) Aspirin, heparin, or both to treat acute unstable angina. N Engl J Med 319:1105–1111

Theroux P, Waters D, Qui S et al. (1993) Aspirin vs. heparin to prevent myocardial infarction during the acute phase of unstable angina. Circulation 88:2045–2048

Coronary Artery Bypass Surgery

Operative Mortality **134**

Complications Associated with CABG **138**

Long-Term Outcomes **139**

Indication for CABG Surgery **140**

Comparison of CABG with Multivessel Angioplasty . . . **141**

References **142**

Each year 300,000 coronary artery bypass grafting (CABG) operations are performed in the United States, 25 % of them in women. Over the past 30 years the patient population undergoing surgery has dramatically changed. In the early 1970s only a few patients (men and women) over the age of 70 years and/or with an ejection fraction less than 50 % were felt to be suitable candidates for CABG. With refinements in technology and increasing operator experience the percentage of high-risk patients significantly rose (Weintraub et al. 1998). In other words, presently there is a much higher percentage of patients with reduced left ventricular function, three-vessel coronary artery disease, diabetes mellitus, and over 70 years of age that undergo CABG than 25 years ago. Due to the increasing number of high-risk patients, operative mortality in men rose from 1 % in 1974 to 2.7 % in 1991 and in women from 1.3 to 5.4 %, respectively. Since coronary artery disease in women generally presents approximately 10–15 years later in life than it does in men women undergoing CABG surgery are significantly older than men. The percentage of men older than 60 years increased from 28.8 % in 1974–1979 to 59.6 % in 1988–1991. The percentage of women over age 60 years was 45.1 % from 1974–1979 and 77.3 % from 1988–1991. Only 3.5 % of men, but 7.3 % of women, were older than 70 years from 1974 to 1979. From 1988 to 1991 it was 24.3 and 38.8 %, respectively.

Operative Mortality

Almost all surgical series document a higher raw operative mortality for women than for men, even in the most recent publications (O'Connor et al. 1993; King et al. 1994; Edwards et al. 1998; Aldea et al. 1999). The relative risk (RR) for women ranges from 1.4 to 4.4. Interestingly, gender differences are most pronounced in the female population with low or intermediate risk for surgery and less in women at high risk for CABG [ejection fraction (EF) <40 %, severe three-vessel coronary artery disease] compared with men with comparable risk. Of note as well is the fact that the percentage of women (like in almost all studies) included in these studies is much lower (20–25 %) than the percentage of men (75–80 %) and that fact alone could cause an erroneous interpretation of data. The following variables, which are discussed in detail later, definitely play an important role with respect to the increased mortality in the female population:

- Smaller body surface area (BSA)
- Smaller size of coronary arteries
- Older age
- High prevalence of diabetes mellitus
- High prevalence of urgent surgery

From a historical perspective operative mortality in women undergoing CABG has been higher than that in men for more than 30 years (Table 7.1). Bolooki et al. (1975) reported an operative mortality of 8 % in women and of 2 % in men. The operative mortality in the Coronary Artery Surgery Study (CASS; Fisher 1982) was 4.5 % in women and 1.9 % in men and strikingly high in women 70 years of age and older (12.3 % in women age >70 years, 2.8 % in women age 35 years). Loop et al. (1983) found that despite the fact that women had better left ventricular systolic function and less extensive coronary artery disease than men, they had a higher in-hospital mortality (2.9 vs 1.3 %); however, almost all studies that statistically adjusted for BSA (on average smaller in women than in men), coronary artery size (on average smaller in women than in men), age (average age in women 66.9 years, in men 63.6 years), and for cardiovascular risk factors (average incidence of diabetes mellitus 15 % in women, 10.6 % in men; hypertension 49 % in women, 33 % in men) gender was *not* an independent risk factor for death. Most studies that did not take these variables into account found that female gender was an independent risk factor for operative mortality. Even recent studies have supported these observations. A prospective study from the Boston Medical Center from 1994 to 1997 (Aldea et al. 1999) in 1743 patients (30 % women) showed that women were older, smaller, had a high incidence of diabetes mellitus, and more often required urgent surgery. Men had a higher likelihood of reduced left ventricular systolic function and of severe three-vessel coronary artery disease. More men than women were smokers. After statistical adjustment for these variables, no gender difference could be detected (mortality rate for women 1.5 %, for men 1.0 %). It is concluded that women – despite refinements in technology and despite increasing operator experience – have a higher risk with CABG surgery; however, the increased risk can be attributed to the older age, smaller body size, and high prevalence of comorbid conditions and not gender; however, in discussing risk of CABG with the patient and the family, it is advisable to include gender in the discussion of risks.

Table 7.1. Gender differences in perioperative mortality of coronary artery bypass surgery. (Adapted from Weintraub 1997)

Authors	Years	Gender	No. of patients	Mortality (%)
Loop et al.(1983)	1967–1980	Women Men	2,245 18,079	2.9 1.3
Bolooki et al.(1975)	1969–1973	Women Men	34 226	8.0 2.0
Douglas et al.(1981)	1973–1979	Women Men	492 2,663	2.2 1.0
Rahimtoola et al.(1993)	1974–1991	Women Men	1,979 6,927	2.7 1.9
Fisher et al.(1982; CASS)	1975–1980	Women Men	1,153 6,258	4.5 1.9
Christakis et al.(1995)	1982–1986	Women Men	1,346 5,988	6.0 3.0
Khan et al.(1990)	1982–1987	Women Men	482 1,815	4.6 2.6
O'Connor et al.(1993)	1987–1989	Women Men	819 2,236	7.1 3.3
Hannan et al.(1989)	1989	Women Men	3,169 9,279	5.4 3.1
Weintraub (1997)	1974–1979	Women Men	Not available NA	1.3 1.0
Weintraub et al.(1998)	1988–1991	Women Men	NA NA	5.4 2.7

NA not available

Variables that play an important role for operative mortality and can be used to calculate risk for CABG are listed in Table 7.2. Of note here as well, female gender is reported as a variable associated with higher mortality. (comparable with reduced LVSF with EF <40 %).

Table 7.2. Preoperative estimation of risk of mortality and stroke in isolated coronary artery bypass surgery (only). (Adapted from Eagle et al. 1999)

Characteristics	Score for mortality	Score for stroke
Age 60–69 years	2	3.5
Age 70–79 years	3	5
Age >80 years	5	6
Women	1.5	
EF <40 %	1.5	1.5
Urgent surgery	2	1.5
Emergency surgery	5	2
Prior CABG	5	1.5
Peripheral vascular disease	2	2
Dialysis or creatinine >2	4	2
COPD	1.5	
Total Score	**Mortality (%)**	**Stroke (%)**
0	0.4	0.3
1	0.5	0.4
2	0.7	0.7
3	0.9	0.9
4	1.3	1.1
5	1.7	1.5
6	2.2	1.9
7	3.3	2.8
8	3.9	3.5
9	6.1	4.5
10	7.7	>6.5
11	10.6	
12	13.7	
12	17.7	
14	>28.3	

CABG coronary artery bypass grafting, *COPD* chronic obstructive pulmonary disease.

It remains unclear why women more often than men undergo urgent surgery. Khan et al. (1990) hypothesized that differences in referral patterns for men and women may be part of the difference: women are referred for angiography later in the course of their disease than men (too late?) and thus undergo CABG later than men (too late?). Furthermore, only women with severe symptoms are referred for CABG in contrast with men who undergo surgery on the basis of a positive stress test (Ayanian and Epstein 1991); however, other factors may play a role as well. For example, it is unknown how many women present too late for evaluation of their disease and how many women refuse surgery; and gender-specific differences cannot be excluded completely, either.

Complications Associated with CABG

Despite the large number of women undergoing CABG each year, there are very few data with respect to intra- and perioperative complications in women. Weintraub et al. (1998) who examined data from 13,625 patients with bypass surgery found no gender difference in the incidence of perioperative myocardial infarction (2–5 %). The most striking difference was a higher incidence of stroke in women in comparison with men (2.7 vs 1.7 %). Several years earlier O'Connor et al. (1993) reported the same observation. Stroke in the perioperative period is associated with a higher mortality. Besides stroke, women are at higher risk than men for postoperative hemorrhage (O'Connor et al. 1993; Weintraub et al. 1998), prolonged mechanical ventilation (Edwards et al. 1998), postoperative renal failure (Edwards et al. 1998), and heart failure (O'Connor et al. 1993; Jacobs et al. 1998; Weintraub et al. 1998). In Bypass and Angioplasty Revascularization (BARI; Jacobs et al. 1998) 9.8 % of women, but only 1.8 % of men experienced congestive heart failure or pulmonary edema. Given the fact that women undergoing CABG have a better left ventricular systolic function than men, heart failure in women is predominately secondary to diastolic and not systolic dysfunction (Judge et al. 1991).

There are essentially no gender-specific data for conduction abnormalities, autonomic dysfunction, sternum dehiscence (frequently seen in obese women), and pneumonia.

Long-Term Outcomes

Although operative mortality is higher in women than in men, there is no gender difference in long-term survival. Loop et al. (1983) reported that after 5 years 90.6 % of women and 93 % of men were still alive. Survival rates after 10 years were 78.6 % for women and 78.2 % for men. Rahimtoola et al. (1993) followed patients for 18 years and found 70 % of women and 73 % of men alive. The small difference in survival was due to the higher operative mortality in women.

However, despite similar long-term survival, more women than men remain symptomatic. Douglas et al. (1981) found that after 21 months only 45 % of women, but 69 % of men were without angina. In the study by Rahimtoola et al. (1993) the reported difference was smaller, but not negligible (79 of women vs 70 % of men were still symptomatic). This study demonstrated also that women have a higher rate of coronary artery bypass graft occlusion than men: after 2 years 23.6 % of grafts in the female population, but only 17.9 % in the male population, were occluded. A possible explanation is the fact that women less often than men receive arterial conduits and in particular less often an internal mammary bypass graft (45 % of women in contrast to 64 % of men). Kirklin et al. (1989) demonstrated a higher survival rate for patients with internal mammary bypass grafts to the LAD, independent of gender (89 vs 71 % after 10 years).

On average, 25 % of saphenous vein grafts are occluded after 5 years and 50 % after 10 years; however, only 10 % of internal mammary grafts are occluded after 10 years.

Due to the fact that women have a lower graft patency rate than men, they need repeat revascularization procedures after CABG more often than after PTCA (Fig. 7.1); however, despite the higher incidence of saphenous vein graft occlusions and less relief of angina, long-term survival does not differ between both genders. Taking into account that women are older and have a higher risk profile, female gender is even an independent predictor of improved long-term survival.

After CABG, women return to work less often than men (41.4 vs 68.5 %). If a patient was working prior to surgery, the likelihood of return to work is higher in both genders, but nevertheless a gender difference remains (60.6 % of women, but 81.6 % of men return to work). Part of the reason for this behavior is the older age of women at the time of surgery and less relief of angina (King et al. 1994).

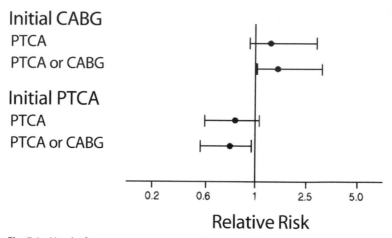

Fig. 7.1. Need of repeat coronary revascularization after coronary artery bypass surgery (*CABG*) in women. (Adapted from Jacobs et al. 1998)

Psychological function, in particular depression and anxiety, is similar for men and women in the early phases after CABG surgery; however, in the longer term, women suffer more depressive symptoms (Almeida et al. 1983) and are less likely to resume pre-operative activities. The higher incidence of comorbid conditions, less social support for women, and the lower likelihood of financial independence play an important role.

Indication for CABG Surgery

There is no doubt that coronary artery bypass surgery is an effective treatment of angina in both genders. Five years after CABG, 75 % of patients, and 10 years after CABG 50 % of patients, are free of angina. Three major studies examined the effect of surgery on survival as well:

- European Cooperative Study
- Veterans Administration (VA) Study
- Coronary Artery Surgery Study (CASS)

However, all studies were conducted prior to routine use of platelet inhibitors and use of an internal mammary graft and before the availability of angioplasty. Based on these studies, surgery was associated with improved survival in the following populations:

- Left main stenosis >70 %
- Three-vessel coronary artery disease and reduced left ventricular systolic function
- Two-vessel coronary artery disease with proximal LAD stenosis and reduced left ventricular systolic function

However, only CASS included women (39 in the medical arm, 37 in the surgery arm). Given the very limited number of women any generalization from these trials is unacceptable. Although the above-mentioned survival benefit with surgery may apply for the general female population as well, it remains unclear whether survival will be improved in older, frail women with serious comorbid conditions.

Whether or not the newer minimally invasive form (LIMA to LAD in a lateral approach and without use of a pump) or the off-pump minimally invasive direct CAB (MIDCAB) on a beating heart but with sternotomy may become alternatives in these high-risk women remains to be seen.

Comparison of CABG with Multivessel Angioplasty

Since 1992 eight studies have compared multivessel angioplasty with CABG in patients suitable for either procedure. In contrast to previous decades, more women were included in these trials (27 vs 15 % in the past); however, only the BARI trial was large enough to permit a subgroup analysis for women (1829 patients, 485 women). Despite the fact that a subgroup analysis was not possible for the other trials, there was a convincing consistency in the clinical results of these trials. The data suggest that this selected patient population is generally at low risk of death or myocardial infarction over the subsequent 3 years and that, except for patients with diabetes mellitus (who showed a survival benefit with CABG over the 5-year follow-up period), neither method of revascularization is associated with a major prognostic advantage.

The incidence of in-hospital mortality was 1.3 % for women and 1.4 % for men, and the rate of NSTEMI 4.7 % for men and 4.6 % for women. Up to 4 years after revascularization women had more angina compared with men regardless of the kind of revascularization; however, at 5 years symptomatic status was not significantly different between genders. Survival curves for men and women after 5 years were virtually superimposed: 87 % of the participating women and 88 % of the men were still alive (Fig. 4.6). Taking into account that women have a higher risk profile, similar extent of CAD and a similar 5-year mortality rate, female gender is even an independent predictor of improved 5-year survival.

● Summary

Women undergoing CABG have a higher operative mortality rate than men; however, the increased risk can be attributed to the older age, smaller body size, and high prevalence of cardiovascular risk factors (particularly diabetes mellitus), and not gender. More women than men require urgent or emergency surgery. Most cases could be prevented if women would seek medical attention earlier and thus be referred for angiography and revascularization at an earlier stage of their disease. Despite a higher operative mortality rate, and despite a higher incidence of perioperative complications, long-term outcome is excellent and does not differ from that in men. Taking into account the higher risk profile in women, similar extent of CAD, and a similar long-term survival rate, female gender is even an independent predictor of improved survival. Therefore, this treatment strategy should be offered to women in need for CABG with anticipation of excellent long-term results; however, in talking to the patient and the family, "gender" as a surrogate marker should be included in the discussion of risks.

References

Aldea GS, Gaudiani JM, Shapira OM et al. (1999). Effect of gender on postoperative outcomes and hospital stays after coronary artery bypass grafting. Ann Thorac Surg 67:1097–1103

Almeida D, Bradford Jm, Wenger NK, King SB, Hurst JW (1983) Return to work after coronary bypass surgery. Circulation 68(supplII):205-213

Ayanian JZ, Epstein AM (1991) Differences in the use of procedures between women and men hospitalized for coronary heart disease. N Engl J Med325:221–225

Bolooki H, Vargas A, Green R, Kaiser GA, Ghahramani A (1975) Results of direct coronary artery surgery in women. J Thorac Cardiovasc Surg 69:271-277

Christakis G, Weisel R, Buth K et al. (1995) Is body size the cause for poor outcomes of coronary artery bypass operations in women? J Thorac Cardiovasc Surg 110:1344–1358

Douglas JS jr, King SB III, Jones EL et al. (1981) Reduced efficacy of coronary bypass surgery in women. Circulation 64:II-11-II-16

Eagle KA, Guyton RA, Davidoff R et al. (1999) ACC/AHA guidelines for coronary artery bypass graft surgery: executive summary and recommendation: A report of the American College of Cardiology/American Heart Association Task Force on Practice Guidelines. Circulation 100:1464–1480

Edwards FH, Carey JS, Grover FL et al. (1998) Impact of gender on coronary bypass operative mortality. Ann Thorac Surg 66:125–131

Hannan EI, Bernard HR, Kilburn HC, O'Donnell JF (1992) Gender differences in mortality rates for coronary artery bypass surgery. Am Heart J123:866-872

Fisher LD, Kennedy JW, Davis KB et al. (1982) Association of sex, physical size and operative mortality after coronary artery bypass in Coronary Artery Surgery Study (CASS). J Thorac Cardiovasc Surg 84:334–341

Jacobs KA, Kelsey S, Brooks MM et al. (1998) Better outcome for women compared with men undergoing coronary revascularization: A report from the Bypass Angioplasty Revascularization Investigation (BARI). Circulation 98:1279–1285

Judge KW, Pawitan Y, Caldwell J et al. (1991) Congestive heart failure symptoms in patients with preserved left ventricular systolic function: analysis of the CASS Registry. J Am Coll Cardiol 18:377

Khan SS, Nessim S, Gray R, Czer LS, Chaux A, Matloff J (1990) Increased mortality of women in coronary artery bypass graft surgery: evidence for referral bias. Ann Intern Med 112:561–567

King KB, Clark PC, Hicks GL (1992) Patterns of referral and recovery in women and men undergoing coronary artery bypass grafting. Am J Cardiol 69:179

King KB, Porter LA, Rowe MA (1994) Functional, social, and emotional outcomes in women and men in the first year following coronary artery bypass surgery. J Womens Health 3:347

Kirklin JW, Naftel DC, Blackstone EH, Pohost GM (1989) Summary of a consensus concerning death and ischemic events after coronary artery bypass grafting. Circulation 79 (Suppl I):81

Kostis JB, Wilson A, O'Dowd K et al. (1994) Sex differences in the management and long-term outcome of acute myocardial infarction. Circulation 90:1715–1730

Loop FD, Golding LR, MacMillan JP et al. (1983) Coronary artery surgery in women compared with men: analyses of risks and long-term results. J Am Coll Cardiol 1:383–390

O'Connor GT, Morton JR, Diehl MJ et al. for the Northern New England Cardiovascular Disease Study Group (1993) Differences between men and women in hospital mortality associated with coronary artery bypass graft surgery. Circulation 88:2104

Rahimtoola SH, Bennett AJ, Grunkemeier GL et al. (1993) Survival at 15 to 18 years after coronary bypass surgery for angina in women. Circulation 88 (part 2):71–78

Weintraub WS (1997) Coronary surgery in women: Outcome, patient selection, access to care. In: Julian DG, Wenger NK (eds) Women and heart disease, vol 11, Dunitz, London, pp 173–181

Weintraub WS, Wenger NK, Jones EL et al. (1998) Changing clinical characteristics of coronary surgery patients: Differences between men and women. Circulation 98:1279–1285

Wenger NK (1990) Gender, coronary artery disease, and coronary bypass surgery. Ann Intern Med 112:557–558

Primary and Secondary Prevention of Coronary Heart Disease

Class I interventions 148

Class II Interventions 161

Class III Interventions 166

References 170

In view of the prevalence of coronary heart disease and the fact that it remains the leading cause of death in the twenty-first century the public health importance of both primary and secondary prevention is obvious. Prevention of even a small percentage of coronary heart disease would not only have a significant impact on reduction in cardiovascular mortality, but also substantially reduce health care costs.

The American College of Cardiology's Bethesda conferences classified all known risk factors into four categories, depending on the causal relationship between factor and disease and the likelihood that intervention strategies reduce the risk (Table 8.1). Gender differences were respected.

On the basis of this scheme incorporating data from prevention studies and their cost-effectiveness, Gaziano et al. (2001) developed a very useful classification of interventions for modifiable risk factors. This classification scheme does not reflect any gender differences; however, the gender-specific importance of each risk factor are discussed in the subsequent chapters.

❶ **Class I interventions (interventions that have been proved to lower risk of coronary heart disease) are:**
- **Smoking cessation**
- **Treatment of hyperlipidemia**
- **Blood pressure management**
- **Cardiac protection with aspirin, beta-blockers, and ACE inhibitors for secondary prevention**

Class II interventions (interventions that are likely to lower risk of coronary heart disease) are:
- **Diabetes mellitus control**
- **Increase of HDL and reduction of triglycerides**
- **Regular physical activity**
- **Weight reduction in obesity**
- **Light to moderate alcohol consumption**

Class III interventions (interventions that potentially lower the risk of coronary heart disease) are:
- **Diet including antioxidant vitamins**
- **Modification of psychosocial factors**

Table 8.1. Cardiovascular disease risk factors and the usefulness of intervention for primary and secondary prevention of coronary artery disease. (Adapted from Gaziano et al. 2001)

Risk factor	Intervention	Primary prevention	Secondary prevention
Smoking	Cessation of smoking	Class I	Class I
↑ Cholesterol	↓ Cholesterol	Class I	Class I
↑ Blood pressure	↓ Blood pressure	Class I	Class I
	Aspirin	Class II	Class I
	ACE inhibitors		Class I
	Beta-blockers		Class I
Diabetes	Diabetes control	Class II	Class II
Low HDL	↑ HDL	Class II	Class I–II
↑ Triglycerides	↓ Triglycerides	Class II	Class II
Physical inactivity	↑ Activity	Class II	Class II
Obesity	Weight reduction	Class II	Class II
	Moderate alcohol consumption	Class II–III	Class II–III
Dietary factors	Improved diet	Class III	Class III

Class I intervention has been proven to be beneficial and cost-effective; *class II* intervention will probably reduce the incidence of events, but data on the benefits, risks, and costs of intervention are limited; *class III* intervention has a potential to reduce risk, but data are incomplete

Class I Interventions

Treatment of Hyperlipidemia

A diet rich in saturated fatty acids, cholesterol, and calories is associated with an increased risk of coronary heart disease. Each reduction of the serum cholesterol level by 1 mg/dl correlates with a reduction in risk by 2–3 %.

To reduce the prevalence of hyperlipidemia the American Heart Association (AHA) and the National Cholesterol Education Program (NCEP) recommend nationwide screening programs for total cholesterol and HDL, regardless of gender. The current guidelines by the NCEP with respect to pharmacological and nonpharmacological interventions are the same for men and women.

Intervention for primary prevention is indicated in individuals with no or one risk factor with serum cholesterol levels >240 mg/dl and LDL >160 mg/dl and with more than two risk factors with cholesterol

Table 8.2. Primary and secondary prevention of dyslipidemia

Primary prevention	Secondary prevention
LDL >160, 0–1 risk factors	
LDL >130, >2 risk factors	
↓	LDL >100
Diet	↓ ↓
LDL >160, >2 risk factors	Diet + statins
LDL >190	
LDL >220, <35 years of age	
LDL >100, Diabetes	
↓	
Diet + statins	

>200 mg/dl and LDL>130 mg/dl. In patients with diabetes mellitus or established coronary heart disease primary therapeutic goal is a LDL <100 mg/dl, followed by an increase of HDL >35 mg/dl and lowering of triglycerides <200 mg/dl (Table 8.2). Both, the AHA and the NCEP, recommend diet as the first-line strategy in primary prevention; however, if treatment goals cannot be achieved by diet alone, medical treatment is indicated, even for primary prevention. In all patients with documented coronary heart disease the combination of diet and therapy with statins are recommended.

Diet

The most important step reducing elevated and maintaining optimal serum lipid- and serum lipoprotein levels is a diet low in cholesterol and low in saturated fatty acids.

Besides weight reduction for obese individuals, the NCEP recommends as a first-line strategy the following diet ("step-1 diet"):

1. <30 % of total calories should be fat
2. <10 % of total calories should be saturated fat
3. >10 % of total calories should be polyunsaturated fatty acids
4. 10–15 % of total calories should be monounsaturated fatty acids
5. <300 mg total cholesterol/day (1 egg=280 mg cholesterol)

Except for minor differences, the AHA diet is the same as the NCEP diet.

If therapeutic goals cannot be achieved after 3 months of a rigorous diet, a further reduction in total cholesterol intake (<200 mg/day) and intake of saturated fatty acids (<7 %) is recommended ("step-2 diet"). For optimal results intensive nutrition counseling by a registered dietitian is indicated.

The major contributors to the intake of saturated fatty acids are the higher-fat red meats (processed meat products, hamburger, veal, lamb, pork), poultry with skin, whole milk, and other dairy products rich in fat (butter, cheese, ice cream, yogurt), and "tropical" fat (coconut and palm oil); the latter are frequently found in nondairy creamers and dairy substitutes (labeled as "cholesterol free"). Commercially available cakes and pastries are rich in saturated fatty acids as well. All saturated fatty acids increase LDL serum levels and therefore they are atherogenic; however, the individual response varies.

Polyunsaturated fatty acids are divided into omega-6 and omega-3 fatty acids. The most common omega-6 fatty acid is linoleic acid (in safflower, sunflower, soybean, and corn oil). Cold-water fish are rich in omega-3 fatty acids (fish oil). Intake of either one of both fatty acids in large amounts reduce serum triglycerides levels. In addition, fish oil is able to reduce platelet aggregation and smooth muscle proliferation, which may play a role in the restenosis rate after percutaneous transluminal angioplasty (PTCA). In contrast to public opinion, fish oil is not able to reduce LDL serum levels and therefore is not a suitable agent in treatment of hypercholesterolemia (regardless of whether it is taken as a drug or eaten in salmon, halibut, or sole). Nevertheless, polyunsaturated fatty acids are useful in primary and secondary prevention of coronary heart disease.

The reduction in serum cholesterol levels with a step-1 diet is approximately 10 % from baseline, and with step 2 an additional 5 %; however, there is a large individual variability in responsiveness ranging from 0 to 25 %. Unfortunately, there are only a few studies evaluating gender differences with respect to nutrition.

The following three studies included a sufficient number of female patients to be meaningful for women: The Finnish Mental Hospital Study (Miettinen et al. 1972) and the Minnesota Coronary Survey Study (Frantz et al. 1989) compared a diet low in saturated fat with "regular" nutrition in 6434 and 4664 women, respectively. The Finnish Mental Hospital Study reported a 34 % reduction in cardiac deaths in the group who received lower dietary saturated fat; however, the difference between the groups did not reach statistical significance. The Minnesota Coronary Survey Study did not find any difference in total and cardiovascular mortality, incidence of myocardial infarction, and ischemia. Unfortunately, both studies were not very well designed and included women with and without coronary heart disease, women with normal cholesterol, and women who did not strictly adhere to the NCEP guidelines.

Hu et al. (1997) demonstrated in a prospectively conducted trial in 80,802 women that replacement of saturated fat with mono- and polyunsaturated fat reduces the risk of coronary heart disease more effectively than reducing overall fat intake.

However, as shown in multiple trials in men and women, substitution of saturated fat with trans-fatty acids (trans-isomer of monounsaturated fat, in most cases elaidic acid, i.e., in margarine and shortening) reduces HDL and increases lipoprotein (a), overall a not desirable effect. Therefore, the Joint Task Force of the American Society for Clinical Nutrition gave the advice that trans-unsaturated fats are less adverse than saturated fats, but less beneficial than polyunsaturated fats.

Bush et al. (1988) found that dietary intervention is less effective in women than in men, but more data have to be obtained.

Given the fact that even in the twenty-first century women have the primary responsibility for food purchasing and preparation, educational efforts for healthy eating have to target the female population.

Medical Therapy of Dyslipidemia

Most guidelines for medical management of dyslipidemia are based on data obtained in men. Most primary and secondary prevention trials included only a relatively small number of women (in most studies the percentage of women varied between 15 and 18 %). Furthermore, women over 65 years and thus women at highest risk for coronary heart disease were frequently excluded from these trials.

Primary Prevention Trials

Only two trials with clinical end points and with drug treatment have included women:
1. Colestipol study (Dorr et al. 1978)
2. Air Force/Texas Coronary Atherosclerosis Prevention (AFCAPS/Tex-CAPS) trial (Downs et al. 1998)

The Colestipol study randomized 1184 women of 2278 individuals to colestipol or placebo, and the AFCAPS/TexCAPS 997 women of 6605 study participants to lovastatin or placebo. Neither in the colestipol study nor in the AFCAPS/TexCAPS trial was a significant difference between the serum- and the control group demonstrated. In contrast to these findings, the West of Scotland Coronary Prevention (WOSCOPS) trial found a 31 % reduction in number of ischemic episodes and nonfatal myocardial infarction in men after 5 years of treatment with pravastatin, which lowered the baseline LDL from 197 to 142 mg/dl. Based on these data and despite the fact that the available studies have limitations, medical therapy for primary prevention of coronary artery disease in otherwise healthy women is not yet recommended. Future research may change the viewpoint, especially since epidemiological studies suggest that lowering of elevated LDL in apparently healthy women reduces the risk of heart disease.

Primary Prevention with Estrogen

The Postmenopausal Estrogen/Progestin Intervention (PEPI) trial (see Chap. 9) clearly demonstrated that estrogen with or without a progestin decreases total cholesterol and LDL and increases HDL in post-menopausal women. Use of estrogen results in a greater increase in HDL cholesterol than use of a statin drug. Because progestins attenuate the positive effects on lipids, therapy with estrogen alone is more effective than a combination therapy. Hormone replacement therapy is a viable option of treating dyslipidemia in postmenopausal women, especially in women with isolated low HDL; however, it has to be taken into account that estrogen increases triglyceride serum levels by 20–25 %.

A combination of estrogen with statins has an additive effect on lipid lowering and is more effective than mono-therapy (Davidson et al. 1997; Darling et al. 1997).

Secondary Prevention Trials with Statins

HMG-Co-A-reductase inhibitors (statins) are the most effective pharmacological agents in lowering LDL (average of 20–40 %, range 25–60 %). They inhibit hepatic cholesterol synthesis and generation of hepatic LDL receptors. All secondary prevention trials in both men and women with HMG-Co-A-reductase inhibitors convincingly documented a clear relationship between lowering of total cholesterol and LDL and a significant reduction in cardiovascular morbidity and mortality.

The 4S-(Scandinavian Simvastatin Survival) trial randomized 4444 patients with coronary heart disease and plasma cholesterol levels between 212 and 312 mg/dl to 20–40 mg Simvastatin or placebo over a time period of 5.4 years. Total cholesterol was lowered by 25 %, LDL by 35 % (from 188 to 122 mg/dl). The HDL increased by 8 %. There was a 32 % reduction in all-cause mortality and 42 % reduction in the risk of coronary death in the simvastatin group. Major coronary events were reduced by 35 % in women (19 % of all patients) and in 34 % in men. Risk reduction seen in the 4S trial was comparable with that of coronary bypass surgery in patients with three-vessel disease and that of beta-blocker therapy after myocardial infarction.

In Cholesterol and Recurrent Events (CARE; Sacks et al. 1996) 576 women and 3683 men with coronary heart disease and with average LDL plasma levels of 139 mg/dl and only mild elevation of total cholesterol (plasma cholesterol level <240 mg/dl) were randomized to 40 mg pravastatin or placebo and followed for 5.4 years. Both men and women treated with pravastatin had significantly lower rates of the primary end-point fatal coronary events or nonfatal myocardial infarction. (Fig. 8.1a). In addition, the need for coronary bypass graft surgery or angioplasty was reduced by 25 % (Fig. 8.1b). Only patients with LDL plasma levels below 125 mg/dl had no benefit. A subgroup analysis for women showed that the effect of pravastatin was greater among women than among men, despite the fact the magnitude of the cholesterol lowering was similar in both genders (cholesterol by 17 %, LDL by 28 %; Table 8.3). There was 43 % risk reduction in the primary end point of fatal coronary events or nonfatal myocardial infarction in women and a 21 % risk reduction in men. The risk of reinfarction was reduced by 57 % in women and by 15 % in men, the need for bypass graft surgery by 39 % in women and by 24 % in men, and the risk of stroke by 59 % in women and by 22 % in men.

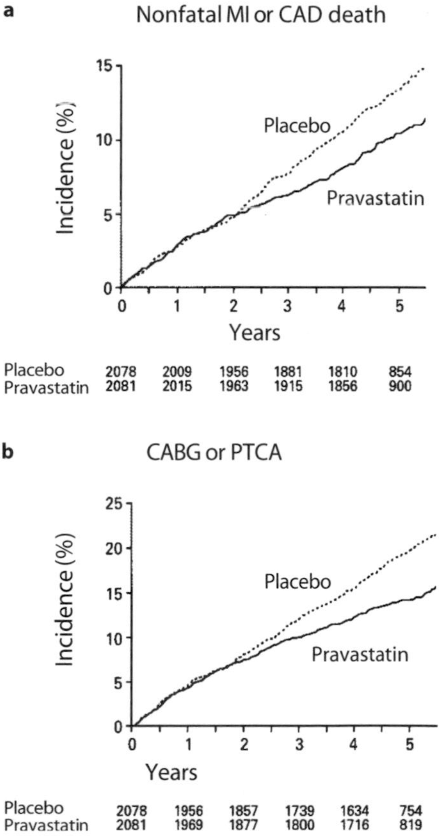

Fig. 8.1a, b. Secondary prevention of coronary artery disease with pravastatin. (From Sacks et al. 1996)

a   Nonfatal MI or CAD death

| Placebo | 2078 | 2009 | 1956 | 1881 | 1810 | 854 |
| Pravastatin | 2081 | 2015 | 1963 | 1915 | 1856 | 900 |

b   CABG or PTCA

| Placebo | 2078 | 1956 | 1857 | 1739 | 1634 | 754 |
| Pravastatin | 2081 | 1969 | 1877 | 1800 | 1716 | 819 |

Table 8.3. Gender differences in secondary prevention of coronary artery disease with pravastatin. (Data from Sacks et al. 1996)

	Women (%)	Men (%)
Cholesterol	17 ↓	17 ↓
LDL	28 ↓	28 ↓
Death or nonfatal myocardial infarction	43 ↓	21 ↓
Reinfarction	57 ↓	15 ↓
CABG	39 ↓	24 ↓
Stroke	59 ↓	22 ↓

CABG coronary artery bypass graft

Given the fact that all end points were significantly lower in women than in men, independent of baseline plasma cholesterol and LDL level and magnitude of lipid lowering effect, statins may have an additional cardioprotective – so far unknown – effect in women. Mechanisms such as platelet inhibition and anti-inflammatory effects are discussed herein (see Chap. 2 and Fig. 2.4).

Secondary Prevention Trials with Medications Other Than Statins

Three major studies evaluated the effect of clofibrate in combination with (no. 1) and without (nos. 2 and 3) nicotinic acid on cardiac mortality:
1. Stockholm Ischemic Heart Disease Trial (103 women, 555 men; Carlson and Rosenhamer 1988)
2. Scottish Society of Physicians Trial (124 women, 717 men; Research Committee of the Scottish Society of Physicians 1971)
3. Newcastle upon Tyne Trial (97 women, 497 men; Groups of Physicians of the Newcastle upon Tyne Region 1971)

The Stockholm Ischemic Heart Disease Trial found a reduction in cardiovascular mortality for the treatment group, but therapy was not blinded and no subgroup analysis for women was performed. The Scottish Society of Physicians Trial and the Newcastle upon Tyne Trial did not find a significant difference between the clofibrate and placebo groups; however, the number of cardiac deaths was small which may explain that a statistical difference could not be demonstrated. Pooled data from both trial showed a lower cardiovascular mortality in the treatment groups.

Gender-specific data with respect to niacin, fenofibrate, and gemfibrozil (fibric acid derivatives) are not available. Since these agents primarily reduce triglycerides (20–40 %) and increase HDL (10–25 %) their main use is as a treatment of hypertriglyceridemia. Their effect on LDL is minimal (0–20 %).

The best way to lower Lp (a) is a combination therapy of estrogen with niacin.

❯ Summary

Statins are very effective in secondary prevention in women. Fibrates are less cardioprotective. Studies with niacin, gemfibrozil, and fenofibrate in women with coronary disease, low HDL (<32 mg/dl), and normal LDL are ongoing.
Unanswered questions are:
1. What is the optimal LDL level in women with coronary heart disease?
2. Which is the best medical therapy (statins, fibrates, or niacin?) in women with low HDL and hypertriglyceridemia?

Treatment of Hypertension

Multiple prospective randomized trials have uniformly demonstrated a reduction in risk of coronary heart disease after 3–6 years of treatment of severe hypertension (systolic blood pressure >180 mmHg, diastolic blood pressure >110 mmHg) in both men and women. Data of medical treatment for mild to moderate hypertension (diastolic blood pressure between 90 and 114 mmHg) are less striking, but a meta-analysis by Collins et al. (1990) nevertheless showed a significant reduction in risk as well:

- A 14 % reduction in the risk of myocardial infarction
- A 21 % reduction in cardiovascular mortality
- A 42 % reduction in the risk of stroke

A recent meta-analysis by Gueyffier et al. (1997) which included approximately 21,000 women and 20,000 men showed a 28–36 % risk reduction in the risk of stroke and major cardiovascular events, but only a trend toward reduced all-cause mortality and cardiovascular death including fatal coronary events. A possible explanation is the fact that the number of elderly women who participated in these trials and who are more likely to show a difference in cardiovascular mortality was small. In other words, the analysis of the data in women had less power to demonstrate reductions in atherosclerotic event rates. Furthermore, aggressive treatment of hypertension may have led to frequent episodes of hypotension with a negative impact on mortality in the young women.

Given the fact that the incidence of coronary heart disease increases with age, studies of older patients are more suitable to ascertain treatment effects. The Swedish Trial in Old Patients with Hypertension (STOP) trial (Dahlof et al. 1993) enrolled patients 70–84 of age. Sixty-three of the patients were women. Medical treatment included metoprolol, atenolol, pindolol, or hydrochlorothiazide vs placebo. The trial was prematurely terminated at 25 months because of a significant reduction in all end points (myocardial infarction, stroke, sudden cardiac death) in the treatment arms. A subgroup analysis for women showed a trend toward more benefit for women, but it did not reach statistical significance.

Not only diastolic hypertension, but also isolated systolic hypertension, is an independent risk factor for coronary heart disease. This form of hypertension is very common in the elderly population. According to the Framingham Study 65 % of women age 65 years and older (vs 57 % of men the same age) have systolic hypertension. The Systolic Hypertension in the Elderly Program (SHEP) trial (SHEP Cooperative Research Group 1991) demonstrated a significant reduction of several end points with treatment of isolated systolic hypertension with chlorthalidone and subsequent addition of a beta-blocker if the target blood pressure was not achieved. Fifty-seven percent of the participating patients were women. There was a 25 % reduction in the risk of coronary heart disease, a 36 % reduction in the risk of stroke, and a 33 % reduction in the risk of myocardial infarction. Even the risk of congestive heart failure was reduced by 49 %. A more recent trial from Europe (Staessen et al. 1999) that randomized 4695 patients age 60 years or older with systolic blood pressure of 160–219 mmHg and diastolic blood pressure less than 95 mmHg to nitrendipine or placebo showed similar reductions in events. There was a 42 % reduction in the risk of stroke and a 32 % reduction in the risk of nonfatal cardiac end points. Cardiovascular and all-cause mortality were lower in the treatment group, but both end points did not reach statistical significance. Results were similar for men and women.

Patients with left ventricular hypertrophy (LVH) are at highest risk of cardiovascular events, according to the Skaraborg Hypertension Project Study (Lindblad et al. 1994), independent of gender. The relative risk (RR) of a myocardial infarction for women with LVH was 2.87 and that of men 2.48.

Table 8.4 shows important studies and the impact of antihypertensive therapy on cardiovascular mortality.

A meta-analysis of several observational studies with thiazides demonstrated that thiazides not only reduce blood pressure but also reduce the risk of hip fractures (by 20 %) due to the fact that thiazide use is associated with a lower renin profile (Cauley et al. 1993; Jones et al. 1995).

Gender-specific data on calcium channel blockers or ACE inhibitors are not yet available.

Three recent major trials (CAPP, INSIGHT, NORDIL) that compared either ACE inhibitor or calcium channel blocker therapy with conventional therapy in both genders did not show any statistically significant difference between treatment groups in the composite end points of cardiovascular events or cardiovascular mortality.

Since ACE inhibitors can cause birth defects, they should be used with caution in women of childbearing age.

Besides medical treatment, multiple non-pharmacological modalities are able to lower blood pressure and should be an essential part of management of hypertension, either as sole form of therapy in patients with mild hypertension or as adjunctive therapy in all other cases.

These lifestyle modifications are:
- Sodium restriction (<6 g sodium chloride)
- Weight reduction if overweight
- Alcohol in moderation (<15 or 15 ml/day)
- Relaxation techniques
- Aerobic physical activity (30–45 min most days of the week; Arroll and Beaglehole 1992; Reaven et al. 1991)
- Adequate intake of potassium (approximately 90 mmol/day)

Table 8.4. Clinical trials in hypertension in women. (Adapted from Bittner and Oparil 1993, 1997)

Study	No. of women	Age (years)	Entry BP	Therapy	Cardiovascular mortality
HDFP (1979–88)	5039	30–69	DB >90	CLTD	No change
Australian Trial (1980)	1257	30–69	DB 95–109	CTZ	–16.9%
EWPHE (1985)	588	Mean age 72	DB 90–119	HCTZ+TMTR	–18%
Coope et al. (1986)	273	60–79	SB >170 DB >105	BDFZ and/ or atenolol	No change
MRC (1985)	8306	35–64	DB 90–109	BDFZ or propranolol	Higher mortality in treated group
MRC (elderly women; 1992)	2560	65–74	SB 160–209 DB<115	Atenolol or HCTZ/Amil	–19%
SHEP (1991)	2690	>60	SB 160–219 DB<90	CLTD +/- Atenolol	–25% CAD –33% MI
STOP (1992)	1025	70–84	SB >180+ DB>90 or DB>105	Multiple	–40%
SHET (1999)	3146	>60	SB 160–210 + DB <95	Nitrendipine ± enalapril, HCTZ	–25%

Amil amiloride, *BDFZ* bendrofluazide, *CLTD* chlorthalidone, *CTZ* chlorothiazide, *DB* diastolic blood pressure, *EWPHE* European Working Party on High Blood Pressure in the Elderly, *HCTZ* hydrochlorothiazide, *HDFP* Hypertension Detection and Follow-up Program, *MRC* Medical Research Council, *SB* systolic blood pressure, *SHEP* Systolic Hypertension in the Elderly Program, *STOP* Swedish Trial in Older Patients with Hypertension, *SHET* Systolic Hypertension in Europe Trial, *TMTR* triamterene, *CAD* coronary artery disease, *MI* myocardial infarction

Lifestyle modification (i.e., weight reduction and physical activity) not only reduces blood pressure but also has a positive impact on several other risk factors that are frequently associated with hypertension such as impaired glucose tolerance, obesity, and dyslipidemia. The Framingham Offspring Study demonstrated that obese women had a sevenfold higher risk of developing hypertension than women with normal body weight. Furthermore, women have more difficulties losing weight than men; therefore, blood pressure control in women by lifestyle modification only is frequently not feasible.

There are few gender-specific data with respect to the effect of physical activity on hypertension; however, studies in both genders show a positive impact of regular exercise on lipid profile, diabetes mellitus, and obesity, and therefore should be recommended in all patients with hypertension.

Moderate alcohol consumption (10–15 g/day or 1–7 drinks/week) is associated with low blood pressure. Alcohol intake of more than 30 mg/day causes hypertension. Therefore the Joint National Committee on Prevention, Detection, Evaluation and Treatment of High Blood Pressure recommends that women not consume more than 15 ml ethanol/day (Moore et al. 1990; Ueshima et al. 1992; Witteman et al. 1990).

Relaxation techniques may be useful in controlling hypertension, although there are conflicting data with respect to the efficacy of this kind of lifestyle modification. Gender-specific data are not available. Interestingly, the Framingham Study found that anxiety in men, but not in women, is associated with the risk of hypertension despite the fact that anxiety is more common in women than in men.

◉ Summary

The prevalence of hypertension increases with age in both genders; however, over age 65 years the prevalence of hypertension is higher in women than in men. Treatment of hypertension lowers the risk of fatal and nonfatal cardiovascular events independent of gender, although data for women age 30–69 years are less compelling than for elderly women (probably due to the fact that these studies did not have enough power to allow conclusive subgroup analyses by gender). First-line therapy for mild hypertension is lifestyle modification. Moderate and severe hypertension requires a combination of nonpharmacological and pharmacological antihypertensive therapy. Isolated systolic hypertension (more frequently seen in elderly women) confers a considerable risk as well and should be treated accordingly. Treatment of hypertension is most important in the presence of left ventricular hypertrophy.

Aspirin

Aspirin leads to a reduced production of thromboxane A2 (a potent promoter of platelet aggregation) by irreversible inhibition of the enzyme cyclooxygenase; hence, aspirin is able to reduce the risk of thrombus formation after plaque rupture. Newer data suggest that aspirin's potent anti-inflammatory properties play an important role in risk reduction as well. There are no known gender differences and in vitro examinations found similar pharmacokinetic properties for both men and women. Low-dose aspirin (80 mg daily) is able to sufficiently inhibit platelet aggregation. High-dose aspirin (>325 mg/day) causes inhibition of prostacyclin as well, overall an unwanted effect since prostacyclin induces vasodilatation and inhibits platelet aggregation as well.

Primary Prevention of CAD with Aspirin

Only four randomized studies have examined the effect of aspirin on the primary prevention of coronary heart disease. All four studies were conducted in men only. Primary prevention trials in women were observational studies with conflicting data. The Nurses' Health Study (87,000 women and a follow-up of 6 years) found a significant reduction in the risk of myocardial infarction (RR=0.75) with the intake of one to six tablets aspirin/day (Manson et al. 1994); however, there was no benefit for women age 50 years or younger. Two other observational studies found no benefit in women; therefore, both the "Preventive Services Task Force" in the United States and the "European Society of Cardiology" in Europe recommend low-dose aspirin for primary prevention only in men. The Women's Health Study (with 40,000 healthy women the largest primary prevention trial in women) will provide more insight into the impact of aspirin in prevention of coronary heart disease in women. Women enrolled in this trial are age 45 years and older and are randomized to 100 mg daily aspirin plus vitamin E every other day, or to placebo. Data are expected in 2005.

Secondary Prevention with Aspirin

In contrast to the conflicting data for primary prevention secondary prevention studies with aspirin clearly show a beneficial effect. A subgroup analysis for women (23 % of the study population) of the Second International Study of Infarct Survival (ISIS-2) trial found a 23 % reduction in cardiovascular mortality and a 49 % reduction in the risk of reinfarction in those women who took 162.5 mg aspirin/day in comparison with those who took placebo. A meta-analysis of 118 studies demonstrated a 35 % reduction in the risk of reinfarction and an 18 % reduction in cardiovascular mortality in all women taking aspirin and at high risk for cardiovascular events (Antiplatelet Trialists' Collaboration 1994). High dosages of aspirin (>325 mg/day) were not more effective than low or medium dosages (75–325 mg/day).

⊘ **Summary**

Women with documented coronary heart disease should be placed on 75–325 mg aspirin/day for secondary prevention of cardiovascular events. Until data from the Women's Health Study are available, and in light of the lack of randomized placebo-controlled trials, aspirin is not indicated for primary prevention in the female population. It could potentially be harmful in cases of a hemorrhagic stroke, a not infrequent occurrence in elderly women, since it may aggravate the bleeding.

Class II Interventions

Physical Activity

A sedentary lifestyle is associated with increased all-cause mortality in both men and women. Prospective observational cohort studies found that women with low physical fitness had a 4.7 relative risk of all-cause mortality compared with women with high physical fitness (O'Toole 1993; Blair et al. 1996). Physical activity not only has a positive impact on most cardiovascular risk factors but also reduces the risk of coronary heart disease and stroke independent of the effect on risk factors. Physical activity could be shown to (a) reduce blood pressure, body weight, and triglycerides, and (b) increase serum HDL levels and insulin sensitivity

There is accumulating evidence that physical activity decreases the risk of various chronic diseases such as colon- and breast cancer, of non-insulin-dependent diabetes mellitus, osteoporosis, and depression.

Until recently, few studies have addressed gender differences in the relationship of habitual physical activity to the risk of CAD. Only 5 of 43 studies published before 1987 included data on women. Furthermore, most of the data were conflicting due to the low number of women enrolled in these trials and different forms of exercise used. These older data report a risk reduction of 60–75 % for women; however, these data appear not reliable given the low number of women and the fact that women age 65 years and older did not participate in these trials.

Over the past decade there have been several primary and secondary prevention trials with a sufficient number of women which are listed below.

Primary Prevention Studies

1. Blair et al. (1993) performed an exercise stress test in 3000 women and 10,000 men at the time of enrollment and after 8 years. Leisure-time physical activity was recorded over this time period. All-cause mortality was elevated in both men and women with low physical fitness (RR=1.5 for men, RR=2.1 for women); however, cardiovascular mortality was only higher for men.

2. LaCroix et al. (1996) found in 1030 women and 615 men age 65 years and older that walking >4 h/week was associated with a significantly higher risk of cardiovascular mortality and a lesser likelihood of admission to the hospital because of cardiovascular illness; however, statistical significance was achieved for women only. Given the high number of women enrolled, the older ages of women, and a focus on the most commonly reported exercise activity, these data appear to be reliable.

3. Recently published data from the Nurses' Health Study (Manson et al. 1999) confirm data from LaCroix et al.: Patients who exercised in the form of fast walking several hours per week had a lower risk of coronary heart disease and stroke. The degree of risk reduction was as high for fast walking as for physical activity of high intensity. Furthermore, women who changed from a sedentary to a physically active lifestyle experienced the same benefit as women who were physically active all their lives.

Secondary Prevention Studies

Two large meta-analyses of randomized clinical trials demonstrated that women after myocardial infarction, who exercise on a regular basis for more than 3 years, have a 25 % reduction in cardiovascular mortality, which is comparable with the benefit of beta-blocker therapy (May et al. 1982; O'Connor et al. 1989).

Further evidence that exercise may slow the progression of atherosclerosis and stabilize coronary lesions is provided by angiographic regression trials (Haskell et al. 1994; Ornish et al. 1990; Schuler et al. 1992). Regression trials examine the impact of lifestyle changes on cardiovascular disease and mortality. Most of these trials include an exercise program (in general moderate-intensity aerobic exercise) as part of a multifactorial intervention. In all studies there was significantly less progression of coronary heart disease in the intervention groups than in the control groups, in women even more so than in men; however, due to the small number of women enrolled the gender difference did not reach statistical significance. Although the use of multifactorial interventions does not permit determination of the unique contribution of physical activity, multivariate regression analysis suggests that physical activity exerts an independent effect on a slower rate of atherosclerotic progression.

Based on these data recent guidelines recommend regular physical activity as an important component of secondary prevention in women with coronary heart disease (Smith et al. 1992; Fuster and Pearson 1996).

The degree of cardiovascular benefit due to physical activity depends on the individual baseline exercise level as well as the exercise intensity, duration, and frequency. The largest benefit is seen in women who shift from a sedentary lifestyle to a moderate amount of regular exercise. Women who participate in regular exercise that is of longer duration or of more vigorous intensity are likely to derive greater benefit; however, an optimal dose of physical activity for maximal cardiovascular risk reduction has yet to be elucidated.

⊘ Summary

Physical activity reduces the risk of coronary heart disease and its progression by 25–50 %. This is even true for women who shift from a sedentary lifestyle to a moderate amount of regular exercise later in life. Benefit can be expected not only from high-intensity activity but also from lower-intensity, shorter-duration activity performed more frequently (i.e., walking >4 h/week in the form of 10-min intervals spread throughout the day).

The following table shows the recommendations of the American Heart Association for physical activity:

Primary prevention:
- Aerobic exercise of moderate to vigorous activity for 30–60 min for 3–4 days/week

Secondary prevention:
- Aerobic exercise of low to moderate activity for 30–60 min for 3–4 days/week

Weight Reduction

The optimal way of weight reduction has not yet been found. It is unclear whether physical activity, diet, behavioral therapies, pharmacological or surgical interventions, or a combination of these modalities, is most effective; however, weight cycling (recurrent weight loss followed by weight gain) appears to be associated with increased cardiovascular morbidity and mortality. Weight loss and weight maintenance should be achieved slowly.

Weight loss has a substantial positive impact on several cardiovascular risk factors:
- Insulin resistance
- Hyperglycemia
- Hypertension
- Hypertriglyceridemia
- HDL

Thus far, there is no effective pharmacological therapy for weight loss. Indirect serotonin antagonists (dexfenfluramine plus phentermine or fenfluramine) are associated with a higher risk of pulmonary hypertension and valvular insufficiency (in particular aortic and mitral regurgitation). Orlistat, which inactivates gastrointestinal lipase, has a moderate effect on weight reduction but increases the risk of colon cancer. Data with respect to sibutramine (which inhibits re-uptake of serotonin and norepinephrine) and leptin analogs are not yet available.

Alcohol

Heavy alcohol consumption not only increases all-cause mortality, but also cardiovascular mortality in both men and women. Light to moderate alcohol consumption (defined as 20–50 g alcohol/day in men and 10–15 g alcohol/day in women, which corresponds to one to nine drinks per week for men and one to three drinks per week for women), however, has been shown to have cardioprotective effects (Gaziano et al. 1993; Stampfer et al. 1988). Most studies evaluating total mortality in men have consistently reported a U-shaped pattern. It is not clear whether the results of these studies may be applicable to women as well. Since women in general have a lower body mass index and a liver metabolism different from that in men, the amount of alcohol that provides a cardiovascular benefit is less in women than in men.

Discussed underlying mechanisms conveyed by light to moderate alcohol consumption are an increase in HDL-, t-PA-, and PAI-I levels, reduction in fibrinogen levels, and a lower tendency for platelet aggregation. The inverse association between light to moderate alcohol intake and CAD is not specific to any type of alcoholic beverage. Although some data suggest that wine is slightly more protective due to a lesser degree of LDL oxidation because of phenols, flavonoids, and tannin found in red wine, other studies have not confirmed these data.

The largest study that has examined the association of alcohol consumption and the risk of coronary heart disease is the Nurses' Health Study. This study demonstrated a statistically significant 40 % reduction in CAD in women consuming 5–14 g alcohol daily (Stampfer et al. 1988). The initially collected but later updated information on alcohol intake showed that the cardiovascular benefit with light to moderate drinking was greatest for women age 50 years or older and/or for women with multiple cardiovascular risk factors; however, women who consumed more than 30 g/day had a 19 % increase in total mortality, primarily due to an increase in death from liver cirrhosis and breast cancer (diseases well known to be caused by heavy alcohol consumption). Whether or not regular light to moderate alcohol intake should be advised remains a difficult question given the potential for addiction and the adverse effects at higher levels of consumption. In addition, our knowledge is based on observational studies only (with the known risk to overestimate benefit), and it is unlikely that randomized trials of alcohol will be performed in the future.

Class III Interventions

Antioxidants

Vitamins E and C

Clinical research data with respect to the association of antioxidant vitamins E and C and risk of coronary heart disease are based on observational studies only, which, again, have a tendency to overestimate benefit. Given the fact that most of these studies were short in duration, in particular the primary prevention studies, the reliability of these data has to be questioned further. We definitely need large-scale randomized trials of sufficient duration. Some studies are underway (most of them are secondary prevention studies), but final results are not expected before 2005.

Basic research has demonstrated that oxidation of lipids and oxidative injury to the vascular wall play an important role in the pathogenesis of atherosclerosis, and that antioxidants may slow down the progression of atherogenesis. In vitro and in vivo studies have shown inhibition of LDL oxidation by the natural antioxidants vitamin C (ascorbic acid), vitamin E (alpha-tocopherol), and, to a lesser degree, by beta-carotene. Besides their antioxidant properties, vitamins C and E are able to inhibit platelet aggregation and to preserve endothelium-dependent vessel relaxation.

The most widely studied antioxidant is vitamin E; however, randomized *primary prevention* studies in women are not yet available. Two primary prevention studies in men, one conducted in malnourished individuals, did not find a risk reduction of coronary heart disease with the intake of vitamin E.

The two largest cohort studies for primary prevention are the Nurses' Health Study (87,000 women, age 34–59 years; Stampfer et al. 1993) and the Iowa Women's Health Study (34,486 women, age 55–69 years; Kushi et al. 1996). The Nurses' Health Study reported a 34 % reduction of nonfatal myocardial infarction and cardiac death for women who consumed more than 100 IU of vitamin E/day in form of a vitamin supplement (in contrast to natural, with diet-ingested vitamin E). In contrast to these data, the Iowa Women's Health Study found an inverse association only for women with vitamin E intake from diet. After statistical adjustment for potential confounders, women in the highest quintile of dietary intake of vitamin E had a 64 % lower risk of CAD mortality than those in the lowest quintile of intake. These conflicting data are potentially caused by the different population studied (women in the Iowa Women's Health Study were older and therefore more suitable to answer the question of a cardioprotective effect of vitamin E) and/or the use of different end points (the Nurses' Health Study examined nonfatal myocardial infarction and coronary death, the Iowa Women's Health Study cardiovascular mortality). Until data from the currently ongoing Women's Health Study (with 40,000 women the largest randomized primary prevention trial) are available, the question of whether vitamin E supplements (600 IU every other day) decreases the risk of CAD remains unanswered. Unfortunately, results will not be available before 2005 and dietary vitamin E will not be examined, either.

Two *secondary prevention* trials were conducted in a randomized fashion. Both trials included men and women, but the number of participating women was small (50 and 312 women, respectively). Both trials did not allow a reliable answer to the question whether vitamin E is beneficial for secondary prevention of coronary heart disease. One of the two studies did not find a statistical significance between the serum- and the control group, and the other study revealed too much disparity in the treatment effects to be conclusive (Stephens et al. 1996). Four large-scale randomized trials with 8000–20,000 women enrolled are underway testing vitamin E alone or in combination with other antioxidants (Table 8.5; Manson et al. 1995) which will provide more insights in the near future.

> **Summary**
> Presently, it remains unclear whether antioxidants (in particular vitamins E and C) reduce the risk and/or the progression of coronary heart disease. Although basic research data clearly suggest that antioxidants play an important role in the pathogenesis of atherosclerosis and may slow down the progression of atherogenesis, data from observational studies in humans are not only conflicting, but also not reliable given a substantial variability in the amount of vitamins used and in form of intake and the short duration of these trials. Results from large-scale randomized trials of sufficient duration for primary and secondary prevention are not yet available. Promising studies, such as the Women's Antioxidant Cardiovascular (WACS) Study and the Heart Protection Study (both examining the effect of vitamin E in combination with vitamin C) are still ongoing. Until these data are available, treatment with these antioxidants cannot yet be advocated.

Table 8-5. Ongoing randomized clinical trials of vitamin E alone or in combination with other antioxidants for secondary prevention of coronary artery disease in women

Study	Antioxidant	Study population	End point(s)
WACS	Vitamin E (600 IU every other day)	8000 women with CAD or ≥3 risk factors	Death, nonfatal MI, CABG or PTCA, stroke
HOPE	Vitamin E (400 IU/day)	9000 women and men with previous MI, PVD, DM, or stroke	Death, nonfatal MI, stroke
GISSI	Vitamin E (300 mg/day)	12,000 women and men with MI <3 months	Total mortality
HPS	Vitamin E (600 IU/day) + beta-carotene (20 mg/day) + vitamin C (50 mg/day)	20,000 women and men with angina, DM, PVD, or stroke	Total mortality

WACS Women's Antioxidant Cardiovascular Study, *HOPE* Heart Outcomes Prevention Evaluation Study, *GISSI* Grupo Italiano per lo Studio della Sopravvivenza nell'Infarcto Miocardio Acuto, *HPS* Heart Protection Study, *CABG* coronary artery bypass grafting, *CAD* coronary artery disease, *MI* myocardial infarction, *PTCA* percutaneous coronary angioplasty, *PVD* peripheral vascular disease, *DM* diabetes mellitus

Beta-carotene

Four randomized *primary prevention* trials were conducted with beta-carotene, three of them only in men; none demonstrated clear evidence of benefit (Hennekens et al. 1996).The Beta-Carotene and Retinol Efficacy Trial (CARET) trial included women but was prematurely discontinued after 4 years because of a projected inability to detect a benefit over the planned funding period and trend toward increased incidence of lung cancer. Furthermore, there was a trend toward increased total and cardiovascular mortality (RR for cardiovascular disease death=1.26).

A subgroup analysis of the Physicians Health Study in 333 men with documented coronary artery disease found a 29 % reduction in risk 12 years after intake of 50 mg beta-carotene every other day. *Secondary prevention* trials in women are not yet available. The WACS Study (600 IU beta-carotene every other day) and the Heart Protection Study are still underway. Results are scheduled to be published in 2005.

⊘ Summary of Primary and Secondary Prevention Interventions

- Dyslipidemia

  A low-fat diet is indicated in all women with dyslipidemia in both primary and secondary prevention. For primary prevention the additional intake of statin drugs is recommended in women with at least two cardiovascular risk factors and LDL >160 mg/dl or in women with diabetes and LDL >100 mg/dl. For secondary prevention statins are indicated in all patients with LDL >100 mg/dl (possibly in all patients with coronary heart disease independent of the LDL level).

- Hypertension

  All women irrespective of age with severe or malignant hypertension should be treated with pharmacological intervention. Women age 65 years and older should receive treatment for each form of hypertension (mild, moderate, severe, malignant, systolic, and diastolic or isolated systolic). Whether or not treatment of mild and moderate hypertension in Caucasian women reduces the risk of coronary heart disease is still a matter of debate.

- Aspirin

  Aspirin is not indicated (yet?) for primary prevention. It is clearly beneficial for secondary prevention. Low-dose aspirin (81 mg once or twice per day) appears to be superior to higher dosages.

- Physical activity

  Physical activity is useful for primary and secondary prevention. Even 4 h/week of walking (even if done in intervals of 10 min) reduces the risk; however, the highest benefit is seen in women who change from a sedentary lifestyle to one with moderate physical activity.

- Weight loss

  Weight loss and weight maintenance should be achieved slowly; weight cycling (recurrent weight loss followed by weight gain) appears to be associated with increased cardiovascular morbidity and mortality.

  Thus far, there is no effective pharmacological therapy without significant side effects for weight loss available yet.

- Alcohol

  Light to moderate alcohol consumption reduces the risk of coronary heart disease; however, alcohol intake of more than 30 g/day is associated with an increase in total mortality, primarily due to an increase in death from liver cirrhosis and breast cancer. Alcohol consumption is not recommended if weight loss is indicated.

▬ Vitamins

Vitamin supplementation for primary or secondary prevention cannot yet be advocated; however, a diet rich in fruits and vegetables lowers the risk of coronary artery disease.

▬ Beta-carotene

Beta-carotene does not reduce the risk and/or progression of coronary heart disease

References

Amery A, Birkenhaeger W, Brixxo P et al. (1985) Mortality and morbidity results from the European Working Party on High Blood Pressure in the Elderly Trial. Lancet I:1349–1354

Antiplatelet Trialists' Collaboration (1994) Collaborative overview of randomized trials of antiplatelet treatment. Part 1: Prevention of death, myocardial infarction, and stroke by prolonged antiplatelet treatment. Br Med J 30:81–106

Arroll B, Beaglehole R (1992) Does physical activity lower blood pressure? A critical review of the clinical trials. J Clin Epidemiol 45:439–447

Bittner V, Oparil S (1993) Hypertension in Women. In: Douglas PS (ed) Cardiovascular health and disease in women. Saunders, Philadelphia, vol 63, p 103

Bittner V, Oparil S (1997) Hypertension. In: Julian DG, Wenger NK (eds) Women and heart disease. Dunitz, London, vol 19, p 311

Blair SN, Kohl HW, Paffenbarger RS et al. (1989) Physical fitness and all-cause mortality: a prospective study of healthy men and women. JAMA 262:2395

Blair SN, Kohl HW, Barlow CE (1993) Physical activity, physical fitness, and all-cause mortality in women: do women need to be active? J Am Coll Netr 12:368–371

Blair SN, Kampert JB, Kohl HW et al. (1996) Influences of cardiorespiratory fitness and other precursors on cardiovascular disease and all-cause mortality in men and women. JAMA 276:205–210

Bush TL, Fried LP, Barrett-Connor E et al. (1988) Cholesterol lipoproteins, and coronary artery disease in women. Clin Chem 1988;34:B60

Byers T. Hardened fats, hardened arteries. N Engl J Med 337:1544–545

Carlson LA, Rosenhamer G (1988) Reduction of mortality in the Stockholm Ischaemic Heart Disease Secondary Prevention Study combined treatment with clofibrate and nicotinic acid. Acta Med Scand 223:405–418

Cauley JA, Cummings SR, Seeley DG (1993) Effect of thiazide therapy on bone mass, fracture and falls. Ann Intern Med 188:666–673

References

Collins R, Peto R, MacMahon S et al. (1990) Blood pressure, stroke, and coronary heart disease. 2. Short-term reductions in blood pressure: overview of randomized drug trials in the epidemiologic context. Lancet 335:827–838

Dahlof B, Lindholm LH, Hansson L et al. (1991) Morbidity and mortality in the Swedish Trial in Older Patients with Hypertension (STOP-Hypertension). Lancet 338:1281–1285

Dahlof B, Hansson L, Lindholm LH et al. (1993) Swedish Trial in Older Patients with Hypertension (STOP-Hypertension) analyses performed up to 1992. Clin Exper Hypertens 15:925–939

Darling GM, Johns JA, McCloud PI, Davis SR (1997) Estrogen and progestin compared with simvastatin for hypercholesterolemia in postmenopausal women. N Engl J Med 337:595

Davidson MH, Testolin LM, Maki KC et al. (1997) A comparison of estrogen replacement, pravastatin and combined treatment for the management of hypercholesterolemia in postmenopausal women, Arch Intern Med 157:1186

Dorr AE, Gunderson K, Schneider JC et al. (1978) Colestipol hydrochloride in hypercholesterolemic patients: effect on serum cholesterol and mortality. J Chron Dis 31:5–14

Downs JR, Clearfield M, Weis S et al. (1998) Primary prevention of acute coronary events with lovastatin in men and women with average cholesterol levels. JAMA 279:1615–1622

Frantz ID, Dawson EA, Ashman PL et al. (1989) Test of effect of lipid lowering by diet on cardiovascular risk: the Minnesota Coronary Survey. Arteriosclerosis 9(1):129–135

Fuster V, Pearson TA (1996) 27th Bethesda Conference: matching the intensity of risk factor management with the hazard for coronary disease events. J Am Coll Cardiol 27:957–1047

Gaziano JM, Manson JE, Ridker PM (2001) Primary and Secondary Prevention of Coronary Heart Disease. In Braunwald E, Zipes DP, Libby P (eds) Heart disease. Saunders, Philadelphia, vol. 32, pp 1040-1065

Gaziano JM, Buring JE, Breslow JL et al. (1993) Moderate alcohol intake, increased levels of high-density lipoprotein and its subfractions, and decreased risk of myocardial infarction. N Engl J Med 329:1829–1834

Groups of Physicians of the Newcastle upon Tyne Region (1971) Trial of clofibrate in the treatment of ischemic heart disease. BMJ 4:767–775

Gueyffier F, Boutitie F, Boissel JP et al. (1997) Effects of antihypertensive drug treatment on cardiovascular outcomes in women and men: a meta-analysis of individual patient data from randomized, controlled trials. Ann Intern Med 126:761–776

Hammond EC, Garfinkel L (1975) Aspirin and coronary artery disease: findings of a prospective study. Br Med J 2:269–271

Haskell WL, Alderman EL, Fair JM et al. (1994) Effects of intensive multiple risk factor reduction on coronary artherosclerosis and clinical cardiac events in men and women with coronary artery disease. Circulation 89:975–990

Hennekens CH, Buring JE, Manson JE et al. (1996) Lack of effect of long-term supplementation with beta-carotene on the incidence of malignant neoplasms and cardiovascular disease. N Engl J Med 334:1145–1149

Hu FB, Stampfer MJ, Manson JE et al. (1997) Dietary fat intake and the risk of coronary heart disease in women. N Engl J Med 337:1491

ISIS-2 (Second International Study of Infarct Survival) Collaborative Group (1988) Randomized trial of intravenous streptokinase, oral aspirin, both, or neither among 17,187 cases of suspected acute myocardial infarction: ISIS-2. Lancet II:349–360

Joint National Committee on Prevention, Detection, Evaluation and Treatment of High Blood Pressure (1997) The Sixth Report of the Joint National Committee on Prevention, Detection, Evaluation and Treatment of High Blood Pressure. Arch Intern Med 157:2413–2446

Jones G, Nguyen T, Sambrook PN, Eismann JA (1995) Thiazide diuretics and fractures: can meta-analysis help? J Bone Mineral Res 10:106–111

Klatsky A, Friedman G, Armstrong M (1986) The relationship between alcoholic beverage use and other traits to blood pressure: a new Kaiser Permanente study. Circulation 73:628–636

Kushi LF, Folsom AR, Prineas RJ et al. (1996) Dietary antioxidant vitamins and death from coronary artery disease in postmenopausal women. N Engl J Med 18:1156–1162

LaCroix AZ, Wienpahl J, White LR et al. (1990) Thiazide diuretic agents and the incidence of hip fracture. N Engl J Med 322:286–290

LaCroix AZ, Leveille SG, Hecht JA et al. (1996) Does walking decrease the risk of cardiovascular disease hospitalizations and death in older adults? J Am Geriatr Soc 44:113–120

Lewis SJ, Mitchell JS, East C et al. (1996) Women in CARE have earlier and greater response to pravastatin on coronary events after myocardial infarction in patients with average cholesterol levels. Circulation 94(8, Suppl. I:69

Lichtenstein AH (1997) Trans-fatty acids, plasma lipid levels, and risk of developing cardiovascular disease: a statement for health care professionals from the American Heart Association. Circulation 95:2588–2590

Lindblad U, Rastam L, Ryden L et al. (1994) Control of blood pressure and risk of first myocardial infarction: the Skaraborg hypertension project. BMJ 308:681–686

Manson JE, Gaziano JM, Spelsberg A et al. (1995) A secondary prevention trial of antioxidant vitamins and cardiovascular disease in women: rationale, design, and methods. Am J Epidemiol 5:255–260

Manson JE, Stampfer MJ, Willet WC et al. (1995) Physical activity and incidence of coronary heart disease and stroke in women. Circulation 91:927

Manson JE, Rich-Edwards JW, Colditz JA et al. (1996) The role of walking in the prevention of cardiovascular disease in women. Circulation 94(Suppl):S339

Manson JE, Hu FB, Rich-Edwards JW et al. (1999) A prospective study of walking as compared with vigorous exercise in the prevention of coronary heart disease in women. N Engl J Med 341:650

References

Manson JE, Stampfer MJ, Colditz GA et al. (1994) A prospective study of aspirin use and primary prevention of cardiovascular disease in women. JAMA 266:521–527

May GS, Eberlein KA, Furberg CD et al. (1982) Secondary prevention after myocardial infarction: a review of the long-term trials. Prog Cardiovasc Dis 24:331–362

Miettinen M, Turpeinen O, Karvonen MJ et al. (1972) Effect of cholesterol-lowering diet on mortality from coronary heart disease and other causes: a twelve year clinical trial in men and women. Lancet II:835–838

Moore RD, Levine DM, Southard J et al. (1990) Alcohol consumption and blood pressure in the 1982 Maryland Hypertension Survey. Am J Hypertens 3:1–7

O'Connor GT, Buring GE, Yusaf S et al. (1989) An overview of randomized trials of rehabilitation with exercise after myocardial infarction. Circulation 80:234–244

O'Toole ML (1993) Exercise and physical activity. In: Douglas PS (ed) Cardiovascular health and disease in women. Saunders, Philadelphia, p 253

Ornish DM, Scherwitz LW, Brown SE et al. (1990) Can lifestyle changes reverse artherosclerosis? Lancet 336:129–133

Paganini-Hil A, Chao A, Ross RK, Henderson BE (1989) Aspirin use and chronic diseases: a cohort of the elderly. Br Med J 299:1247–1250

Reaven PD, Barrett-Connor E, Edelstein S (1991) Relation between leisure-time physical activity and blood pressure in older women. Circulation 83:559–565

Research Committee of the Scottish Society of Physicians (1971) Ischemic heart disease: a secondary prevention trial using clofibrate. BMJ 4:775–784

Sacks FM, Pfeffer MA, Moye et al. (1996) The effect of pravastatin on coronary events after myocardial infarction in patients with average cholesterol levels. N Engl J Med 335:1001–1009

Scandinavian Simvastatin Survival Study Group (1994) Randomized trial of cholesterol lowering in 4.444 patients with coronary heart disease: The Scandinavian Simvastatin Survival Study (4 S). Lancet 344:1383–389

Schuler G, Hambrecht R, Schlierf G et al. (1992) Regular physical exercise and low-fat diet: effects on progression of coronary artery disease. Circulation 86:1–11

SHEP Cooperative Research Group (1991) Prevention of stroke by antihypertensive drug treatment in older persons with isolated systolic hypertension: final results of the Systolic Hypertension in the Elderly Program (SHEP). JAMA 265:3255–3264

Smith SC, Blair SN, Criqui MH et al. (1992) Preventing heart attack and death in patients with coronary disease. Circulation 86:1–11

Stampfer MJ, Colditz GA, Willett WC et al. (1988) A prospective study of moderate alcohol consumption and the risk of coronary disease and stroke in women. N Engl J Med 319:267–273

Stampfer MJ, Hennekens CH, Manson JE et al. (1993) Vitamin E consumption and the risk of coronary disease in women. N Engl J Med 328:1444–1449

Stephens NG, Parsons A, Schofield PM et al. (1996) Randomized controlled trial of vitamin E in patients with coronary disease: Cambridge Heart Antioxidant Study (CHAOS). Lancet 347:781–786

Summary of the Second Report of the National Cholesterol Education Program (NCEP) Expert Panel on Detection, Evaluation, and Treatment of High Blood Cholesterol in Adults (Adult Treatment Panel II) (1993) Expert Panel on Detection, Evaluation and treatment of high blood cholesterol in adults. JAMA 269:3015

Ueshima H, Ozawa H, Baba S et al. (1992) Alcohol drinking and high blood pressure: data from a 1980 national cardiovascular survey of Japan. J Clin Epidemiol 45:667–673

West of Scotland Coronary Prevention Study Group (1998) Influence of pravastatin and plasma lipids on clinical events in the West of Scotland Coronary Prevention Study (WOSCOPS). Circulation 97:1440–1445

Witteman JCM, Willette WC, Stampfer MJ et al. (1990) Relation of moderate alcohol consumption and risk of systemic hypertension in women. Am J Cardiol 65:633–637

Women's Health Study Research Group (1992) The Women's Health Study: rationale and background. J Myocardial Ischemia4:30–40

Hormone Replacement Therapy

Hormone Replacement Therapy
and Prevention of Coronary Heart Disease 176

Observational Studies for Primary
and Secondary Prevention. 177

Randomized Primary Prevention Trials 178

Randomized Secondary Prevention Trials 180

Clinical Implications of Hormone
Replacement Therapy 185

Biological Mechanisms of Hormone
Replacement Therapy 193

References 198

Hormone Replacement Therapy and Prevention of Coronary Heart Disease

Coronary heart disease continues to be an infrequent disease in pre-menopausal women, even in women with diabetes mellitus; however, after menopause (the time when estrogen production decreases) the preva-lence of coronary heart disease in women increases with increasing age and reaches that of men by age 75 years. Women with premature menopause (<35 years of age) regardless of etiology (either natural or af-ter ovariectomy) have a twofold higher risk of coronary heart disease (Wenger et al. 1993). These findings led to the conclusion that estrogens are cardioprotective and play a major role for the low prevalence of car-diovascular disease in pre-menopausal women; however, the role of estro-gen (and other hormones) in the pathogenesis of coronary heart disease is still under investigation.

Thirty-three epidemiological studies found that hormone replace-ment therapy (HRT) reduces the risk of coronary heart disease by 35–50 % (Bush et al. 1987; Barrett-Connor and Bush 1991; Henderson et al. 1991; Grady et al. 1992;Grodstein et al. 1997); however, all but one study were ob-servational studies which are associated with several drawbacks:

1. In contrast to randomized, placebo-controlled observational studies, they have a tendency to overestimate the benefit of the therapy.
2. Observational studies are associated with "selection bias artifact."
3. Patients who participate in observational studies are generally healthy, lead a healthy lifestyle (non-smoker, regular exercise, not overweight, low-fat diet), and are compliant with their medications (note that it could be shown that patients compliant with their med-ications have 40–60 % reduction in the risk of coronary heart disease even while taking placebo).

Indeed, most of the participating women in the above-mentioned studies were young and relatively healthy (no or very few comorbid conditions), had no or very few risk factors, and lead a healthy lifestyle, all of which could have had an impact on the positive outcome of HRT. Furthermore, even after statistical adjustment for these variables, other unknown fac-tors may have influenced the data; therefore, a direct relationship between HRT and a reduced risk of coronary heart disease remains hypothetical until data from randomized placebo-controlled studies are available. On the other hand, the available data are useful. They not only allow insights in the effects of HRT on risk factors and delineate risk and benefits of hormone substitution, but also shed light on the impact of hormones on development and progression of coronary heart disease.

Observational Studies for Primary and Secondary Prevention

Over the past 25 years 33 studies have examined the effect of HRT on *primary prevention* of coronary heart disease. Thirty-two of the 33 studies were not randomized and only 14 of the 33 studies were conducted in a prospective manner. There was only one prospective randomized trial and that trial did not include more than 84 women. In this study there was a mild, but not significant reduction, in the risk of myocardial infarction with HRT (RR=0.3).

Thus far, the largest epidemiological trial with respect to HRT and risk of coronary artery disease (CAD) is the still ongoing Nurses' Health study (Stampfer et al. 1986, 1991). Besides HRT, the investigators examined the impact of diet, physical activity, and lifestyle changes on the risk of coronary heart disease as well. Since 1976, 121,700 nurses age 30–55 years without known heart disease and without diabetes mellitus agreed to fill out a questionnaire every other year. Since 1988 interim results have been published. The Nurses' Health study and (in concert with 12 other studies) found a significant reduction of coronary heart disease with regular HRT (average RR=0.6), even after statistical adjustment for risk factors such as age, hypertension, and smoking. Cardioprotection was seen even in women age 75 years and older and for women at low and high risk of coronary heart disease; however, the highest reduction in cardiovascular mortality (49 %) was found in women with at least one cardiovascular risk factor (smoking at the time of evaluation, hyperlipidemia, hypertension, diabetes mellitus, genetic disposition for coronary heart disease, obesity with a body mass index >29) and the least reduction was seen in women without risk factors (RR=0.89). Five years after discontinuation of the drug, no clinical benefit was seen. Ten years after continued hormone intake, the beneficial effects were less pronounced than at the beginning of therapy, most likely due to the fact that there was a 43 % increase in death from breast cancer.

Important observational primary prevention studies with HRT are listed in Table 9.1 (Nurses' Health study is listed under Stampfer et al. 1986)

Table 9.1. Important observational studies for primary prevention of coronary heart disease with hormone replacement therapy

Study	Year	Relative risk
Stampfer et al.	1986	0.30*
Bush et al.	1987	0.34*
Henderson et al.	1988	0.54*
Folsom et al.	1995	0.74
Criqui et al.	1988	0.81
Wilson et al.	1985	1.94

*$p < 0.05$

Despite the fact that all studies point in the same direction and, on average, demonstrate a 50 % reduction in the risk of CAD with HRT, these data have to be interpreted with caution given the fact that these were observational studies only.

Up to 1998 all *observational secondary prevention* studies reported an even greater benefit with HRT than the primary prevention trials. In these trials there was a 50–90 % reduction in cardiovascular mortality (see Table 9.2).

Randomized Primary Prevention Trials

Presently, two major *randomized primary prevention studies* are underway: the Women's Health Initiative (WHI) trial (see WHI website) and the Women's International Study of Long-Duration Oestrogen After the Menopause (WISDOM) in Europe. Final results of both trials are expected in 2005 and 2008, respectively; however, the estrogen-plus-progestin component of the Women's Health Initiative trial was already prematurely discontinued because of an increased risk of breast cancer and cardiovascular events (Writing Group for the WHI 2002).

Table 9.2. Important observational studies for secondary prevention of coronary heart disease with hormone replacement therapy

Study	Year	Reduction (%)	End point(s)
Brett et al.	1995	47	Death from coronary cause
Newton et al.	1995	50	Death from coronary cause
Nachtigall et al.	1992	74	Death from coronary cause
Bush et al.	1991	82	Death from coronary cause
Henderson et al.	1991	66	Death from coronary cause
Cooperative Study Group	1986	82	Death, stroke, retina infarction
Sullivan et al.	1990	90	Death

The hormone subgroup of the WHI trial an NIH-sponsored study in the United States is the first large prospectively conducted randomized double-blind primary prevention trial. A total of 27,348 healthy women age 50–79 years (out of 160,000) are randomized to either estrogen (patients with history of hysterectomy, 45 % of all participating women) or estrogen with medroxyprogesterone acetate (women without hysterectomy) or placebo. Follow-up was scheduled to be 8.5 years, but the estrogen-plus-progestin component was discontinued after 5.2 years. Contraindications for enrollment are/were a history of endometrial or breast cancer, pulmonary embolism, or deep vein thrombosis. Primary end point is total mortality (not cardiac mortality!), and secondary end point nonfatal myocardial infarction.

On 31 May 2002, after a mean of 5.2 years of follow-up, the data and safety monitoring board recommended stopping the trial of estrogen plus progestin vs placebo (16,608 patients) because the test statistic for invasive breast cancer exceeded the stopping boundary for this adverse effect and the global index statistic supported risks exceeding benefits. All-cause mortality was not affected during the trial. Estimated hazard rations [HRs; nominal 95 % confidence interval (CI)] were reported as follows: coronary heart disease 1.29 (CI 1.02–1.63); breast cancer 1.26 (CI 1.00–1.59); stroke 1.14 (CI 1.07–1.85); and pulmonary embolism 2.13 (CI 1.39–3.25).

Corresponding heart rate (HR) for the composite end point for total cardiovascular disease (arterial and venous disease) was 1.22 (CI 1.09–1.36). Only the risk of colorectal cancer (HR 0.63) and endometrial cancer (HR 0.83), and the risk of hip fracture (HR 0.66), was reduced with continuous combined HRT (Fig. 9.3).

The other large randomized primary prevention study is the WISDOM study in Europe, including the United Kingdom which enrolled approximately 50 % of 34,000 women. The study design is similar to that of the WHI and has a 10-year follow-up. The primary outcome is combined fatal or nonfatal myocardial infarction and recurrent ischemia.

Randomized Secondary Prevention Trials

In sharp contrast to the data from observational trials are published results from three randomized trials. In particular, the Heart and Estrogen/Progestin Replacement Study (HERS) completely changed our view of HRT for prevention of subsequent cardiovascular events (Hulley et al. 1998). It was the first clinical trial that evaluated in a randomized fashion whether the continuous combined regimen of estrogen plus progestin reduced cardiovascular mortality or nonfatal myocardial infarction in postmenopausal women with established coronary artery disease. 2763 women (mean age, 67 years) were randomized to either 0.625 mg conjugated equine estrogen plus 2.5 mg medroxyprogesterone acetate (none of the women had a history of hysterectomy) or placebo. Patients with a cardiac event in the last 6 months, serum triglyceride level greater than 300 mg/dl, heart failure New York Heart Association class III and IV, uncontrolled hypertension or diabetes, HRT over the last 3 months, history of deep vein thrombosis, uterine or breast cancer or any other fatal disease were excluded. After 4 years there was no significant difference in the primary coronary heart disease outcome (death from coronary cause and nonfatal myocardial infarction) between the HRT- and the placebo group. There were 179 events in the HRT group and 182 in the placebo group (Table 9.3). This null effect was present despite a significant improvement in lipid profile (10 % increase in HDL, 11 % reduction in LDL). Secondary cardiovascular outcomes such as need for revascularization (either PTCA or CABG) and incidence of unstable angina did not differ either (Fig. 9.1). In subsequent analyses a significant time trend not only of coronary ar-

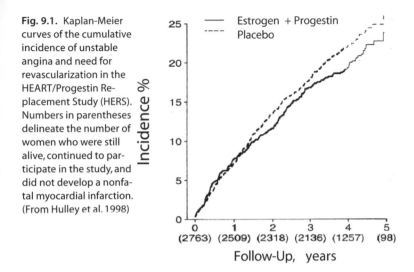

Fig. 9.1. Kaplan-Meier curves of the cumulative incidence of unstable angina and need for revascularization in the HEART/Progestin Replacement Study (HERS). Numbers in parentheses delineate the number of women who were still alive, continued to participate in the study, and did not develop a nonfatal myocardial infarction. (From Hulley et al. 1998)

Table 9.3. Cardiovascular events in the Heart and Estrogen/Progestin Replacement Study (HERS). (From Hulley et al. 1998)

	E+P (n=1380)	Placebo (n=1381)	Relative risk	p value
Total cardiovascular events	179	182	0.99	0.91
Death from coronary cause	70	59	1.20	0.31
Nonfatal myocardial infarction	122	134	0.92	0.50

E+P=0.625 mg conjugated equine estrogen plus 2.5 mg medroxyprogesterone acetate/day

tery events, but also for the thromboembolic complications could be seen suggesting early harm and possible later benefit: in the first year of treatment there were 52 % more cardiac events in the HRT group, in year 4 and 5 there were 25 % fewer cardiac events; there were 34 thromboembolic complications in the HRT group in contrast to 12 events in the placebo group that decreased over the 4 year period (Fig. 9.2). The implication was that a net benefit for coronary heart disease events would have been observed with longer duration of treatment.

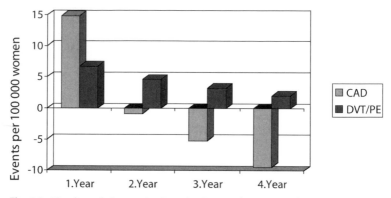

Fig. 9.2. Number of deep vein thrombosis or pulmonary embolism (*DVT/PE*) in comparison to cardiac events (*CAD*) in women receiving HRT. (From Herrington 2001)

The HERS II study (Grady et al. 2002) was an unblinded follow-up study of HERS to determine whether the risk reduction observed in later years of HERS persisted. Ninety-three percent of the women who participated in HERS (2321 women) consented to follow-up. The majority of the women (89 %) taking hormones (which were 45 % of women assigned to HRT at the initiation of the trial) reported taking oral conjugated estrogens (0.625 mg/day) plus 2.5 mg of medroxyprogesterone acetate. Only 8 % of women who had been assigned to placebo began taking HRT after treatment assignment was unblinded. The primary outcome was nonfatal myocardial infarction and coronary heart disease death. Secondary cardiovascular events were coronary revascularization, hospitalization for unstable angina or congestive heart failure, nonfatal ventricular arrhythmia, sudden death, stroke or transient ischemic attack, and peripheral vascular disease. After 6.8 years (or an additional 2.7 years) there were no significant decreases in rates of primary coronary heart disease and secondary cardiovascular events in comparison with placebo. The unadjusted relative hazard (RH) for coronary events in HERS II was 1.00 (95 % CI 077–1.29). In essence, lower rates of coronary heart disease events among women in the hormone group in the final years of HERS did not persist during additional years of follow-up. The authors concluded that post-menopausal hormone therapy should not be used to reduce the risk for coronary heart disease events in women with coronary heart disease.

Of interest as well is the fact that the overall increase in the risk of venous thromboembolism and biliary tract surgery in HRT users persisted. Of considerable importance also, the risk of fracture was not decreased with HRT.

How can these data be explained? The increased risk for coronary heart disease events might be due to prothrombotic, proinflammatory, or proarrhythmic effects of hormones (Grady et al. 2000).

It is well known that estrogen has a prothrombotic effect that has a negative impact on women at high risk for thromboembolic complications (i.e., women with obesity, women with factor V Leiden); thus, coronary events may reflect arterial thrombosis causing increased cardiovascular morbidity and mortality.

Recently, it was shown that estrogen increases high sensitivity C-reactive protein (hs-CRP) and thus has a proinflammatory effect as well. Since inflammation plays an important role in development and progression of CAD, this mechanism may also contribute to estrogen's hazardous effect.

Another possible reason for the increased event rate may be due to the fact that the trial was conducted with a combination of estrogen with a progestin and not with estrogen alone and/or due to the kind of progestin (in this case medroxyprogesterone acetate). It has been suggested that progestins offset the cardiovascular benefit of estrogen. In addition, animal research data and data from the Postmenopausal Estrogen/Progestin Interventions (PEPI) trial demonstrated that the combination of estrogen with medroxyprogesterone acetate has the least beneficial effect on vascular reactivity, on progression of coronary artery plaques, and on the lipid profile than a combination of estrogen with micronized progestin or than estrogen alone; however, preliminary results from the WHI (2001) randomized trial of the effect of hormone therapy revealed an increased risk of cardiovascular events during the first years of follow-up among women treated with estrogen alone as well. In addition, the Coronary Drug Project secondary prevention trial found also an early increase in nonfatal myocardial infarction and coronary heart disease death in men randomized to a high dose of conjugated estrogen (Wenger et al. 2000).

The Estrogen Replacement (ERA) study reports similar results as HERS and HERS II (Herrington et al. 2000). The ERA examined the effect of HRT on coronary atherosclerosis in 309 postmenopausal women with angiographically verified coronary heart disease. Fifty percent of the participating women had a history of myocardial infarction and 50 % a history of percutaneous transluminal coronary angioplasty (PTCA). Women who at least had a 30 % lesion of their coronary angiogram were included in the study and randomized to either 0.625 mg equine conjugated estrogen, estrogen plus 2.5 mg medroxyprogesterone acetate, or placebo. Primary end point was a new atherosclerotic plaque and/or progression of the existing lesion(s). Angiographic follow-up was, on average, after 3.2 years. In contrast to placebo, women on HRT had a significant improvement in their lipid profile (reduction of LDL by 10–15 %, increase of HDL by 14–18 %). Despite these findings, there was no difference in the mean minimal coronary artery diameter on repeat coronary angiograms between the three groups and, although not part of the study design, there was no difference in the clinical outcome of myocardial infarction, ischemia, or need for revascularization.

Further data will derive from a small secondary prevention trial called Women's Hormone Intervention Secondary Prevention Pilot (WHISP) study which was conducted from October 1999 to December 2000 and randomized women with a history of a myocardial infarction to estrogen, estrogen plus a progestin, and placebo.

◉ Summary

Despite the fact that estrogen has multiple anti-atherogenic effects (including a positive alteration of the lipid profile, antioxidative properties, propensity for vasodilatation) estrogen replacement therapy and in particular HRT (estrogen plus a progestin) is associated with an early increased risk of cardiovascular events and no reduction of events with long-term treatment in women with and at risk for coronary heart disease. The underlying mechanisms are most likely prothrombotic and proinflammatory effects of progestins (and probably estrogen as well) that outweigh any effects of estrogens on atherogenesis and vasodilatation; therefore, postmenopausal HRT should *not* be used for primary and secondary prevention.

Whether or not primary prevention with *estrogen alone* may reduce the risk of coronary artery disease has to be determined, but preliminary results suggest increased risk as well.

Continuation of HRT should be based on established noncoronary benefits and risks and patient preference.

Clinical Implications of Hormone Replacement Therapy

Approximately 38 % of postmenopausal women in the United States use HRT. In 2000, 46 million prescriptions were written for Premarin (conjugated estrogen) and 22.3 million prescriptions for Prempro (conjugated estrogen plus medroxyprogesterone acetate). Premarin is the second most frequently prescribed medication in the United States (Fletcher and Colditz 2002). Although the U.S. Food and Drug Administration approved HRT only for relief of postmenopausal symptoms and prevention of osteoporosis, women take estrogens for various (unproven) reasons including prevention of Alzheimer's disease, coronary heart disease, and stroke.

The most widely studied estrogen with respect to cardiovascular disease is equine conjugated estrogen (dosage 0.625–0.9 mg/day). The most common dosage is 0.625 mg/day. Young women frequently need higher dosages than 0.625 mg/day to overcome postmenopausal symptoms.

Table 9.4. Equivalent hormone dosages

Estrogen preparations
0.625 mg conjugated equine estrogen (Premarin)
1.0 mg micronized estradiol (Estrace)
0.625 mg piperazine estrone sulfate (Ogen)
Transdermal estradiol
0.05 mg estradiol/24 h, changed once/week (Climara) or twice/week (Estraderm)
Estrogen plus progestin
0.625 mg conjugated estrogen plus 2.5 mg medroxyprogesterone acetate daily (Prempro in a single tablet) or 5 mg medroxyprogesterone acetate days 1–14 (Premarin plus Provera)
1.0 mg micronized estradiol plus 0.5 mg norethindrone (Activelle)
Transdermal estrogen plus progestin
0.025 mg estradiol plus 0.125 mg norethindrone (CombiPatch)

Table 9.5. Contraindications to hormone replacement therapy

Absolute
Vaginal bleeding of unknown etiology
Pregnancy
Breast or endometrial cancer
Deep vein thrombosis or history of thromboembolic events
Questionable
History of breast or endometrial cancer
Relative
Uterine leiomyomas
Endometriosis
Migraine headaches
Thrombotic events secondary to oral contraceptives
Cholelithiasis
Liver disease
Hypertriglyceridemia
Severe hypertension

Few data are available for other forms of HRT, such as transdermal applications. Since transdermal applications do not have any significant impact on lipid metabolism and the coagulation system, they may have different effects and side effects than oral preparations. It is, for example, possible that transdermal applications do not increase the risk of thromboembolic complications.

The most commonly used estrogen medications and estrogen-plus-progestin medications are listed in Table 9.4. Contraindications for HRT are listed in Table 9.5.

Combination Therapy

A combination of estrogen with a progestin is indicated in all women
without a hysterectomy, since estrogen alone increases the risk of endometrial dysplasia by 33 % and of uterus cancer by 6 % after 3 years of
intake (The Writing Group for the Postmenopausal Estrogen/Progestin
Interventions Trial 1995). According to current literature the progestin
therapy only protects against endometrial cancer and has no other beneficial effects. It even may be harmful and responsible for most of the
proinflammatory responses seen in the HERS trial and estrogen plus
progestin component of the WHI trial.

Furthermore, progestins administered alone have androgenic effects
and a negative impact on lipid parameters: They decrease HDL, and increase LDL and total cholesterol. In addition, they increase glucose intolerance; however, data form the PEPI trial (a 3-year, multicenter, randomized, double-blind, placebo-controlled trial that assessed the impact of
HRT on lipids, lipoprotein(a), fibrinogen, insulin, and blood pressure)
demonstrated that at the time of combination therapy of estrogen with a
progestin estrogen's beneficial impact on lipid parameters is able to overcome the negative modification of the lipid profile by the progestin: all
treatment groups (0.625 mg of equine conjugated estrogen plus 10 mg
medroxyprogesterone acetate in a cyclic manner, 0.625 mg of equine conjugated estrogen plus 2.5 mg medroxyprogesterone acetate in a continuous manner, 0.625 mg of equine conjugated estrogen plus 200 mg micronized progesterone in a cyclic manner, or 0.625 mg of equine conjugated estrogen alone) were associated with a decrease in LDL (up to 15 %)
and increase in HDL (up to 15 %). The estrogen alone therapy, however,
had the highest and the combination with medroxyprogesterone acetate
the least lipid-lowering effect (Table 9.6). Estrogen alone was the only
form of HRT that was able to reduce fibrinogen. Since the Framingham
Heart Study it is well known that elevated fibrinogen levels are an independent risk factor for myocardial infarction and stroke.

Risk of Breast Cancer with HRT

Up to 2002 data with respect to the risk of breast cancer due to HRT were
conflicting. The PEPI trial did not find an increased risk after 3 years of
treatment; however, the duration of the trial may have not been long

Table 9.6. Effect of hormone replacement therapy on lipoprotein level (percent increase or decrease). (Modified from The Postmenopausal Estrogen/Progestin Intervention Trial 1995; and Douglas 2001)

	Placebo	E alone	E+P cyclic	E+P continuous	E+MP
TC	−11	−20	−36	−36	−20
LDL	−11	−37	−46	−43	−38
HDL	−3	+14	+4	+3	+11
TG	−4	+15	+14	+13	+15
Lp(a)	0	−17	−26	−20	−22

E conjugates estrogen 0.625 mg daily, *E+P cyclic* 0.625 mg conjugates estrogen/day plus 10 mg medroxyprogesterone acetate/day for 12 days/month, *E+P continuous* E+2.5 mg P/day, *E+MP* E+200 mg micronized progestin/day for 12 days/month, *TC* total cholesterol, *TG* triglycerides

enough to ascertain risk. Latest data from the Nurses' Health study report a 43 % increase of death due to breast cancer after 10 year of HRT. The Office of Technology Assessment Study reports an RR of 1.35, and the European Position Paper on Hormone Replacement and Menopause an RR of 1.2–1.4 after 8–15 years of therapy. The highest risk was found for women age 60 years or older (RR=1.71), at a time when HRT is most often used for prevention of osteoporosis (Colditz et al. 1995; Grodstein et al. 1997). The increased risk of breast cancer in these trials was independent of a genetic disposition. A recent meta-analysis of all epidemiological studies showed that there was a mild increase in risk after 5 years of hormone intake that continuously increased with duration of use (Table 9.7). Five years after discontinuation of HRT, the risk was the same as without HRT, regardless of duration of treatment and dosage (Dupont and Page 1991; Steinberg et al. 1991). Most cases of breast cancer during HRT were found in the early stages of cancer and from a histological standpoint these tumors were not very aggressive.

As mentioned previously, these data were derived either from observational studies or studies of short duration.

The first large randomized primary prevention trial of postmenopausal hormones and duration of more than 3 years – the WHI –

Table 9.7. Hormone replacement therapy and risk of breast cancer. (Modified from Fleming 1999)

Hormone replacement therapy	Cumulative incidence of breast cancer
Example: Women between 50 and 70 years	
Never	45 cases/1000 women
5 years	2 additional cases (CI 1–3)
10 years	6 additional cases (CI 3–9)
15 years	12 additional cases (CI 5–20)
Example: Women >70 years	
Never	63 cases/1000 women
20 years	75 cases/1000 women
Took hormones for 20 years, no intake for previous 5 years	63 cases/1000 women

CI confidence interval

discontinued prematurely the estrogen plus progestin component of the trial because of a significant increased risk of invasive breast cancer (hazard ratio 1.26; confidence interval 1.00–1.59) that did not begin until 3 years of treatment. The increased risk of the estrogen/progestin combination means that in 10,000 women taking the drug for 1 year, there will be eight more invasive breast cancers. Results were remarkably consistent in subgroup analyses suggesting that there is no subgroup not being affected by this outcome. The data and safety monitoring board did not recommend stopping the estrogen alone component of this trial in women with hysterectomies; therefore, estrogen alone may be safer than the combination of estrogen with a progestin. Despite the fact that these results can be applied for the dosing regimen "0.625 mg of equine conjugated estrogen plus 2.5 mg medroxyprogesterone acetate in a continuous manner" only, other regimens point in the same direction (Chen et al. 2002; Ross et al. 2000; Schairer et al. 2000).

Given these results, it is indicated that clinicians stop prescribing this combination for long-term use. The purpose of HRT in healthy women is to prevent disease. These data demonstrate that the opposite is happening, even if the absolute risk is low.

Risk of Ovarian Cancer with HRT

Until recently, the association between menopausal HRT and ovarian cancer was unclear. Most retrospective studies found no association, and in those studies that showed an increased risk the association was not significant. A large, prospective study from 2001 was the first to report a significant twofold increased risk of ovarian cancer mortality among long-term users of *estrogen* replacement therapy (Rodriguez et al. 2001). Limited data are available on HRT with estrogen and a progestin and the risk of ovarian cancer. The Breast Cancer Detection Demonstration Project (BCDDP), a nationwide breast cancer screening program in 44,241 postmenopausal women, was the first to examine the risk of ovarian cancer with different regimens of hormone replacement in a large prospective cohort (Lacey et al. 2002). It found that women who used estrogen-only replacement therapy, particularly for 10 years or more, were at significantly increased risk of ovarian cancer. The relative risk (RR) was on average 1.6 (95 % CI 1.2–2.0). Relative risks for 10–19 years and 20 years or more were 1.8 (95 % CI 1.1–3.0) and 3.2 (95 % CI 1.7–5.7), respectively. In the study by Lacey et al. the risk of ovarian cancer was not increased among women who used short-term-estrogen–progestin regimens; however, the latter data are based only on a small number of women and a lesser duration of follow-up than data from the estrogen-alone regimen. Nevertheless, based on these findings it is recommended to weigh the risks and benefits of estrogen replacement therapy on an individual basis, noting that risks of estrogen-only therapy now include ovarian cancer (Noller 2002).

Risk of Endometrial Cancer with HRT

Each year 2 of 100,000 postmenopausal women develop endometrial cancer. After 2–4 years of estrogen-replacement therapy (estrogen alone!) the risk increases three- to fivefold. The combination estrogen/progestin is not associated with an increased risk (Grady et al. 1995). Risk increases with longer duration of use and with higher dosages of estrogen. Even several years after discontinuation of estrogen there is still a slightly higher risk of endometrial cancer. Estrogen-induced endometrial carcinomas in general are small and well differentiated, which makes treatment and outcome favorable.

Risk of Deep Vein Thrombosis and Thromboembolic Events

Hormone replacement therapy stimulates hepatic production of coagulation factors and increases fibrinolytic activity; thus, HRT is associated with an increased risk of deep vein thrombosis (DVT) and pulmonary embolism (Fig. 9.3). Previous studies have reported that the annual incidence of DVT is 16/100,000 women and the annual incidence of pulmonary embolism is 5/100,000 women; however, no appreciable increase in risk of DVT or pulmonary embolism was found in past users of HRT. Although the absolute risk of DVT or pulmonary embolism is small, the RR is significant. In the Oxford Study the RR for spontaneous DVT and pulmonary embolism was 3.5 and in the Puget-Sound study 3.3 (Daly et al. 1996; Jick et al. 1996). The Nurses' Health study did not report a higher incidence of DVT, but it did report an increased risk of pulmonary embolism (RR=2.1; Grodstein et al. 1996a). The highest risk occurs in the first year of treatment, regardless of whether taken orally or in the form of a transdermal patch.

As outlined above, the estrogen-plus-progestin component of the WHI that was prematurely discontinued because of increased risk of breast cancer also showed an increased risk of pulmonary embolism with a HR of 2.13 (CI 95 % 1.39–3.25).

Also of great concern is an increased risk of myocardial infarction with initiation of treatment. The WHI reported an HR for nonfatal myocardial infarction of 1.32 (95 % nominal CI 1.02–1.72). These data confirm previous findings from observational studies: The Nurses' Health study and the Puget-Sound study found an increased risk of myocardial infarction in the first year of treatment. In the Nurses' Health study this increased risk was true only for women with coronary heart disease (RR=2.1), but in the Puget-Sound study it was true even in young healthy women (RR=1.39). In contrast to the WHI, the risk in the Nurses' Health and in the Puget-Sound study diminished over time and was present 1–2 years after beginning HRT (Nurses' Health study RR=1.1; Puget-Sound study RR=0.61).

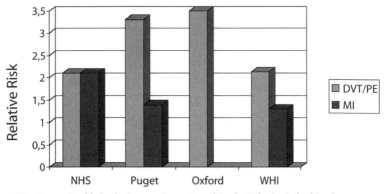

NHS = Nurses Health Study, Puget = Puget Sound Study, Oxford = Oxford Study,
WHI = Women's Health Initiative, DVT = Deep vein thrombosis, MI = Myocardial infarction
PE= Pulmonary Embolism

Fig. 9.3. Early risk of cardiac events or deep vein thrombosis/pulmonary embolism
with hormone replacement therapy. *MI* myocardial infarction. (From Writing Group
for the Women's Health Initiative Investigators 2002)

Discussed mechanisms are, again, a proinflammatory and prothrombotic effect of estrogen and progestin as well.

Estrogen and High Sensitivity C-reactive Protein

It has been shown that plasma levels of high sensitivity C-reactive protein (hs-CRP) increase with HRT (Fig. 9.4). Women enrolled in the WHI and taking HRT (both estrogen alone and in combination with progestin) had a twofold-higher mean hs-CRP level than women on placebo. Similar data were reported form the MONICA study in Germany and from the PEPI trial. In PEPI HRT resulted in an overall 85 % increase in hs-CRP that was sustained for 36 months. It is well known that elevated hs-CRP levels are associated with an increased risk of cardiac events including sudden cardiac death. These findings correlate well with the increased risk of myocardial infarction seen in the HERS trial, the WHI, the Puget Sound study and in the Nurses' Health study.

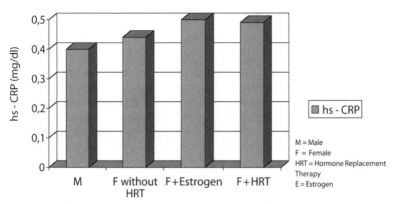

Fig. 9.4. High sensitivity C-reactive protein (hs-CRP) levels by gender and hormone replacement therapy. (Adapted from Ridker 1999)

◆ Summary

Hormone replacement therapy is associated with multiple risks: It increases the risk of deep vein thrombosis and pulmonary embolism, and in the first year of treatment the risk of a myocardial infarction. Hormone replacement therapy with estrogen alone may increase the risk of ovarian cancer after 10 years of intake. The combination of estrogen with a progestin is associated with a higher incidence of invasive breast cancer that begins after 3 years of treatment. Estrogen replacement therapy is also associated with an increased risk of endometrial cancer; however, this risk is essentially eliminated with the combination of estrogen plus progestin.

Biological Mechanisms of Hormone Replacement Therapy

Lipids and Antioxidant Effects of Estrogen

Estrogen increases HDL cholesterol (10–15 %) and apoprotein A-I levels. It reduces total cholesterol (10–15 %), LDL cholesterol (10–15 %), and Lp(a) levels. The reduction in LDL cholesterol is most likely secondary to an increased density of LDL receptors in the liver and thus increased LDL catabolism. Although estrogen increases VLDL and triglycerides, a negative

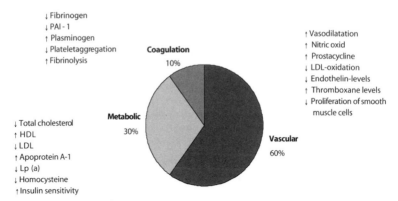

↓ Fibrinogen
↓ PAI - 1
↑ Plasminogen
↓ Plateletaggregation
↑ Fibrinolysis

Coagulation
10%

↑ Vasodilatation
↑ Nitric oxid
↑ Prostacycline
↓ LDL-oxidation
↓ Endothelin-levels
↑ Thromboxane levels
↓ Proliferation of smooth
muscle cells

Metabolic
30%

↓ Total cholesterol
↑ HDL
↓ LDL
↑ Apoprotein A-1
↓ Lp (a)
↓ Homocysteine
↑ Insulin sensitivity

Vascular
60%

Fig. 9.5. Potential positive biological effects of hormone replacement therapy (percentage reflects estimated contribution to total benefit)

impact on the incidence or progression of coronary heart disease could not yet be demonstrated.

The combination therapy of estrogen with a progestin is associated with lesser reduction in total cholesterol and Lp-a and a lesser increase in HDL than a therapy with estrogen alone. Reduction in LDL is not affected by the combination treatment.

Oxidized LDL plays an important role in development and progression of atherosclerosis. The 17-β estradiol inhibits LDL oxidation. The HDL promotes cholesterol transport from the vessel wall to the liver and thus cholesterol degradation. It is estimated that in the presence of HDL and estrogen LDL oxidation is reduced by 50 % (Sack et al. 1994).

Glucose Metabolism

Despite the fact that oral contraceptives impair glucose tolerance, postmenopausal HRT has no negative impact on glucose metabolism. Some authors even report a reduction in insulin resistance associated with obesity.

Hemostasis

Elevated factor VII- and fibrinogen levels have to be shown to be independent risk factors for myocardial infarction (and stroke). The Atherosclerosis Risk in Communities Study and the PEPI trial demonstrated that estrogen replacement therapy decreases fibrinogen levels. Since oral estrogen undergoes first-pass clearance in the liver, it has effects on hepatic metabolism, including the production of the procoagulant factors VII, IX, and X. Estrogen replacement therapy increases factor-VII levels, whereas HRT (estrogen plus progestin) seems to have no significant effect on factor VII.

Plasminogen activator inhibitor 1 (PAI-1) is the primary inhibitor of tissue plasminogen activator (t-PA). High levels of circulating estrogen are associated with reduced PAI-1 levels and increased fibrinolytic activity. These effects are attenuated with combined HRT.

Vascular Reactivity

Increased vascular reactivity plays an important role in the pathogenesis of acute coronary syndromes and acute myocardial infarction. Attenuation of vasoconstriction may lead to a reduced incidence of myocardial ischemia and episodes of plaque rupture. Estrogen promotes vasodilatation by several mechanisms:
- Increased production of nitric oxide
- Increased production of prostaglandins
- Calcium antagonistic effects
- Reduction in endothelin-1 and acetylcholine-induced vasoconstriction

These effects are estrogen-receptor dependent. Estrogen receptors can be found in smooth muscle cells and in endothelial cells (Gilligan et al. 1994; Mendelsohn and Karas 1999; Reis et al. 1994; Weiner et al. 1994).

Impact on Markers of Inflammation

Recent data point out that inflammation plays an important role in the development and progression of atherosclerosis. On one hand, estrogen inhibits acute-phase reactants (i.e., intercellular adhesion molecules and monocytes), and on the other hand, it is associated with increased levels of hs-CRP. The WHI demonstrated that hs-CRP is the strongest predictive marker of myocardial infarction, need for coronary revascularization, stroke, and cardiovascular death in apparently healthy postmenopausal women, even in women with normal LDL cholesterol levels. Given the increased incidence of myocardial infarction and stroke with initiation of HRT, the proinflammatory effects of HRT most likely overshadow the inhibition of acute phase reactants.

◗ Summary

Estrogen has major anti-atherogenic effects, e.g., the following:
1. Improved endothelial-dependent vascular reactivity due to increased production of nitric oxide and prostaglandins
2. Favorable effects on the lipoprotein profile
3. Reduced LDL oxidation
4. Reduction of thrombotic potential and increased fibrinolytic activity due to reduction of PAI-1 levels and reduction in fibrinogen

However, estrogen's prothrombotic and proinflammatory actions overshadow these and other not mentioned cardioprotective effects and thus disprove the hypothesis that estrogen or HRT reduces the risk of coronary heart disease.

Selective Estrogen Receptor Modulators

Given the increased risk of endometrial, breast, and possible ovarian cancer with HRT, there has been interest in developing drugs that mimic the beneficial effects of estrogen in bone and cardiovascular and nervous system but antagonize carcinogenic actions. Selective estrogen receptor modulators (SERMs) are synthetic compounds that act as agonists in some tissue (i.e., bone) and as antagonists in other tissue (i.e., breast) depending on which estrogen receptor subtype predominates; therefore, these drugs are not associated with an increased risk of uterus or breast cancer.

Two commonly used SERMS are tamoxifen and raloxifene. Both have agonistic actions in uterus (tamoxifen more than raloxifene) and bone (raloxifene more than tamoxifen) and antagonistic actions in breast. Although both tamoxifen and raloxifene are used primarily for prevention of breast cancer and osteoporosis, both have potential to reduce cardiovascular events. Tamoxifen could be shown to decrease total cholesterol, and to reduce the incidence of hospitalizations for cardiac symptoms and the risk of a fatal myocardial infarction (Walsh et al. 1998; Khovidhunkit and Shoback 1999). Animal studies demonstrated that raloxifene reduces total and LDL cholesterol, Lp(a) and fibrinogen levels, but has no effect on atherosclerotic plaques. The HDL cholesterol, triglycerides, and hs-CRP are not affected by raloxifene.

The first clinical data with respect to raloxifene and cardiovascular events were derived from the Multiple Outcomes of Raloxifene Evaluation (MORE) trial. The MORE trial is a multicenter randomized placebo-controlled trial designed to determine whether 3 years of raloxifene reduces the risk of fracture in postmenopausal women with osteoporosis. A total of 7705 women were randomized to either placebo or 60 mg/day or 120 mg/day raloxifene. Secondary end points were the incidence of cardiovascular disease and the incidence of breast cancer. Although only 2 % of the participating women had a history of coronary heart disease, 2738 of the 7705 women had one or several cardiovascular risk factors. The prevalence of diabetes in this trial was 2.5 %. There was a significant 40 % reduction in cardiovascular events in the raloxifene groups. The reduction of risk was even more pronounced in women who had a previous myocardial infarction (55 % reduction). Furthermore, raloxifene reduced the incidence of breast cancer by 65 %; however, this was restricted to estrogen-receptor positive tumors; on the other hand, the risk of DVT was 3.1 times higher in women assigned to raloxifene.

Since the MORE trial was not designed to answer the question of cardiovascular outcome, data has to be obtained from a randomized clinical trial with a primary coronary heart disease end point. In 2006 data from the Raloxifene Use for The Heart (RUTH) trial will be available. The RUTH is multicenter randomized placebo-controlled trial in 10,000 postmenopausal women with risk factors for coronary heart disease designed to determine whether 60 mg raloxifene daily has an impact on cardiovascular risk factors and eventually on the combined end point death from coronary cause, nonfatal myocardial infarction, and hospitalization for acute coronary syndrome. Secondary end points are the incidence of unstable angina, stroke, breast cancer, fractures, and thromboembolic events. Enrollment has been completed, but even preliminary data are not yet available.

Until more studies (in particular the RUTH trial) are completed, the use of raloxifene should be limited to the prevention and treatment of osteoporosis. At this point it is still uncertain whether SERMs will play a role in primary and secondary prevention of coronary heart disease.

Soy Protein

Soy protein contains isoflavones, predominately genistein and daidzein. Isoflavones are labeled as phytoestrogens or plant estrogens since they have weak estrogenic and antiestrogenic effects. In postmenopausal women with very low endogenous estrogen levels phytoestrogens bind to the estrogen receptor in some tissues and induce estrogen-like effects. Isoflavones taken in form of soy protein only (not in form of a isoflavone-rich soy extract or in red clover) have LDL-lowering effects as well as the ability to inhibit LDL oxidation. In addition, there is a modest cholesterol-lowering effect but perhaps only in women with elevated cholesterol levels. The HDL does not change with soy protein intake. The U.S. Food and Drug Administration approved foods that contain at least 25 g/day of soy protein and are part of a diet low in saturated fat and cholesterol for prevention of cardiovascular disease. Data from large randomized trial are not yet available.

> **◗ Summary**
> At this time, there is no clinical trial evidence that tamoxifen, raloxifene, or soy protein prevent coronary heart disease.

References

Barrett-Connor E, Bush TL (1991) Estrogen and coronary heart disease in women. JAMA 265:1861–1867

Barrett-Connor E, Grady D, Sashegyi A et al. (2002) Raloxifene and cardiovascular events in osteoporotic postmenopausal women: four-year results from the MORE (Multiple Outcomes of Raloxifene Evaluation) randomized trial. J Am Med Assoc 287:847–857

Bergkvist L, Adami HO, Persson I et al. (1989) Prognosis after breast cancer diagnosis in women exposed to estrogen and estrogen-progesterone replacement therapy. AM J Epidemiol 130:221–228

Blumenthal RS, Zacur HA, Reis SE, Post WS (2000) Beyond the null hypothesis – Do the HERS results disprove the estrogen/coronary heart disease hypothesis? Am J Cardiol 85:1015–1017

Brett KM, Madans JH (1995) Long-term survival after coronary heart disease: comparisons between men and women in a national sample. Ann Epidemiol 5:25–32

Bush TL (1991) Long-term effect of estrogen use on cardiovascular death in women. AHA Meeting, November 1991, Orlando/FL

Bush TL, Barrett-Connor E, Cowan LD et al. (1987) Cardiovascular mortality and non-contraceptive estrogen use in women: results from the Lipid Research Clinics Program follow-up study. Circulation 75:1102–1109

Chen CL, Weiss NS, Newcomb P et al. (2002) Hormone replacement therapy in relation to breast cancer. J Am Med Assoc 287:734–741

Colditz GA, Hankinson SE, Hunter DJ et al. (1995) The use of estrogens and progestins and the risk of breast cancer in postmenopausal women. N Engl J Med 332:1589

Collaborative Group on Hormonal Factors in Breast Cancer (1997) Breast cancer and hormone replacement therapy: collaborative reanalysis of data from 51 epidermiologic studies of 52,705 women with breast cancer and 108,411 women without breast cancer. Lancet 350:1047–1059

Collins P, Rosana G, Sarrel PM et al. (1995) Estrogen attenuates acetylcholine-induced coronary arterial constriction in women but not in men with coronary heart disease. Circulation 92:24–30

Criqui MH, Suwarez L, Barrett-Connor E et al. (1988) Postmenopausal estrogen use and mortality. Am J Epidemiol 128:606–614

Cummings SR, Eckert S, Krueger KA et al. (1999) The effect of raloxifene on the risk of breast cancer in post-menopausal women: Results from the MORE (Multiple Outcomes of Raloxifene Evaluation) trial. JAMA 281:2189

Cushman M, Legault C, Barrett-Connor E et al. (1999) Effect of postmenopausal hormones on inflammation-sensitive proteins: The postmenopausal estrogen/progestin interventions (PEPI) study. Circulation 100:717

Daly E, Vessey MP, Hawkins MM et al. (1996) Risk of venous thromboembolism in users of hormone replacement therapy. Lancet 348:977

Dupont WD, Page DL (1991) Menopausal estrogen replacement therapy and breast cancer. Arch Intern Med 151:67–72

Fleming KC (1999) Hormone replacement therapy: practical prescribing. In: Charney P (ed) Coronary artery disease in women. American College of Physicians, Philadelphia, p 294Folsom AR, Mink PJ, Sellers TA et al. (1995) Hormonal replacement therapy and morbidity and mortality in a prospective study of postmenopausal women. Am J Publ Health 85:1128–1132

Fletcher SW, Colditz GA (2002) Failure of estrogen plus progestin therapy for pre-vention. J Am Med Assoc 288:366–368

Folsom AR, Mink PJ, Sellers TA et al. (1995) Hormonal replacement therapy and mor-bidity and mortality in a prospective study of postmenopausal women. Am J Publ Health 85:1128–1132

Gerhard M, Ganz M (1995) How do we explain the clinical benefits of estrogen? Cir-culation 92:5

Gilligan DM, Quyyumi AA, Connon RO III (1994) Effects of physiological levels of es-trogen on coronary vasomotor function in postmenopausal women. Circula-tion 89:2541–2551

Grady D, Rubin SM, Petitti DB et al. (1992) Hormone therapy to prevent disease and prolong life in postmenopausal women. Ann Intern Med 117:1016–1037

Grady G, Gebretsadik T, Kerlikowske K et al. (1995) Hormone replacement therapy and endometrial cancer risk; A meta-analysis. Obstet Gynecol 85:304–313

Grady D, Hulley SB, Furberg C (1997) Venous thromboembolic events associated with hormone replacement therapy. JAMA 278:477

Grady D, Wenger NK, Herrington D et al. (2000) Postmenopausal hormone therapy increases risk for venous thrombembolic disease. The Heart and Estrogen/Prog-estin Replacement Study. Ann Intern Med 132:689–696

Grady D, Herrington D, Bittner V et al. for the HERS RESEARCH GROUP (2002) Cardio-vascular disease outcomes during 6.8 years of hormone therapy: Heart and Es-trogen/Progestin Replacement Study Follow-up (HERS II). J Am Med Assoc 288:49–57

Grady D, Wenger NK, Herrington D et al. (2000) Postmenopausal hormone therapy increases risk for venous thrombembolic disease: the Heart and Estrogen/prog-estin Replacement Study. Ann Intern Med 132:689–696

Grodstein F, Stampfer MJ, Goldhaber SZ et al. (1996a) Prospective study of exoge-nous hormones and risk of pulmonary embolism in women. Lancet 348:983

Grodstein F, Stampfer MJ, Manson JE et al. (1996b) Postmenopausal estrogen and progestin use and the risk of cardiovascular disease. N Engl J Med 332:1589

Grodstein F, Stampfer MJ, Colditz GA et al. (1997) Postmenopausal hormone therapy and mortality. N Engl J Med 336:1769

Grodstein F, Manson JE, Stampfer MJ et al. (1999) Postmenopausal hormones and re-currence of coronary events in the Nurses' Health Study (abstract). Circulation 100:I-871

Henderson BE, Paganini-Hill A, Ross RK. (1988) Estrogen replacement therapy and protection from acute myocardial infarction. Am J Obstet Gynecol 159:312–317

Henderson BE, Paganini-Hill A, Ross RK (1999) Decreased mortality in users of estro-gen replacement therapy. Arch Intern Med 151:75–78

Herrington DM (1999) The HERS trial results: Paradigms lost? Ann Intern Med 131:463

Herrington DM, Beboussin KB, Brosnihan KB et al. (2000) Effects of estrogen replace-ment on the progression of coronary-artery atherosclerosis. N Engl J Med 343:522–529

References

Herrington DM (2001) What about estrogens now? Curr J Rev 10 (2)]

Hulley S, Grady D, Bush T et al. (1998) Randomized trial of estrogen plus progestin for secondary prevention of coronary heart disease in postmenopausal women. JAMA 280:605–613

Jick H, Derby LE, Myers MW et al. (1996) Risk of hospital admission for idiopathic venous thromboembolism among users of postmenopausal oestrogens. Lancet 348:981

Khovidhunkit W, Shoback DM (1999) Clinical effects of raloxifene hydrochloride in women. Ann Intern Med 130:431

Lacey JV Jr, Mink PJ, Lubin JH et al. (2002) Menopausal hormone replacement therapy and the risk of ovarian cancer. J Am Med Assoc 288:334–341

Lobo RA: Hormones, hormone replacement therapy, and heart disease. In Douglas PS (ed): Cardiovascular Health and Disease In Women. Philadelphia, WB Saunders, 1993, p 153

Love RR, Newcomb PA, Wiebe DA et al. (1990) Effects of tamoxifene therapy on lipid and lipoprotein levels in postmenopausal patients with node-negative breast cancer. J Natl Cancer Inst 82:1327

Mendelsohn ME, Karas RH (1999) The protective effects of estrogen on the cardiovascular system. N Engl J Med 340:1801

Miller BA, Ries LAG, Hankey BF et al. (eds) (1992) Cancer Statistics Review: 1973–89. National Cancer Institute, Washington DC, NIH pub no 92, p 2789

Mosca L, Barret-Connor E, Wenger NK et al. (2001) Design and methods of the Raloxifene Use for The Heart (RUTH) Study. Am J Cardiol 88:392–395

Nachtigall LE, Nachtigall RH, Nachtigall RD et al. (1979) Estrogen replacement therapy. Part II: A prospective study in the relationship to carcinoma and cardiovascular and metabolic problems. Obstet Gynecol 54:74–79

Nachtigall M, Smilen SW, Nachtigall RD et al. (1992) Incidence of breast cancer in a 22-year study of women receiving estrogen-progestin replacement therapy. Obstet Gynecol 80:827–830

Newton KM (1995) Estrogen replacement therapy and prognosis after first myocardial infarction [Abstract]. AHA Meeting, November 1995, San Diego/CA

Noller KL (2002) Estrogen replacement therapy and risk of ovarian cancer. J Am Med Assoc 288:368–369

Pamela S, Douglas PS (2001) Coronary artery disease in women. In: Braunwald E, Zipes DP, Libby P (eds) Heart disease. Saunders, Philadelphia

Reis SE, Gloth ST, Blumenthal RS et al. (1994) Ethinyl estradiol acutely attenuates abnormal coronary vasomotor responses to acetylcholine in postmenopausal women. Circulation 89:52–60

Rich-Edwards JW, Manson JE, Hennekens CH et al. (1995) The primary prevention of coronary heart disease in women. N Engl J Med 332:1758–1766

Ridker PM, Hennekens CN, Rifai N et al. (1999) Hormone replacement therapy and increased plasma concentration of C-reactive protein. Circulation 100:713

Rodriguez C, Patel AV, Calle EE, Jacob EJ, Thun MJ (2001) Estrogen replacement therapy and ovarian cancer mortality in a large prospective study of US women. J Am Med Assoc 285:1460–1465

Ross RK, Paganini-Hill A, Wan P, Pike M (2000) Effect of hormone replacement therapy on breast cancer: estrogen versus estrogen plus progestin. J Natl Cancer Inst 92:328–332

Rutqvist LE, Mattsson A (1993) Cardiac and thromboembolic morbidity among postmenopausal women with early-stage breast cancer in a randomized trial of adjuvant tamoxifene: The Stockholm Breast Cancer Study Group. J Natl Cancer Inst 85:1398

Sack MN, Rader DJ, Cannon RO III (1994) Oestrogen and inhibition of oxidation of low-density lipoproteins in postmenopausal women. Lancet 343:269–270

Schairer C, Lubin J, Troisi R et al. (2000) Menopausal estrogen and estrogen-progestin replacement therapy and breast cancer risk. J Am Med Assoc 283:485–491

Stampfer MJ, Willett WC, Colditz GA et al. (1986) A prospective study of postmenopausal estrogen therapy, and coronary heart disease. N Engl J Med 313:1044–1049

Stampfer MJ, Colditz GA, Willett WC et al. (1991) Postmenopausal estrogen therapy and cardiovascular disease: ten-year follow-up from the Nurses' Health study. N Engl J Med 325:756

Steinberg KK, Thacker SB, Smith JC (1991) A meta-analysis of the effect of estrogen replacement therapy on the risk of breast cancer. JAMA 265:1985–1990

Sullivan JM, Vander Zwaag R, Hughes JP et al. (1990) Estrogen replacement and coronary artery disease: effect on survival in postmenopausal women. Arch Intern Med 150:2557–2562

Sullivan JM, El-Zeky F, Vander Zwaag R, Ramanathan KK (1995) Estrogen replacement therapy after coronary artery bypass surgery: Effect on survival. Circulation 345:669

The American-Canadian Cooperative Study Group (1986) Persantine Aspirin Trial in cerebral ischemia. Part III: Risk factors for stroke. Stroke 17:12–18

The Writing Group for the PEPI Trial (1995) Effects of estrogen or estrogen/progestin regimens on heart disease risk factors in postmenopausal women. The Postmenopausal Estrogen/Progestin Interventions (PEPI) trial. JAMA 273:199–208

Walsh BW, Kuller LH, Wild RA et al. (1998) Effects of raloxifene on serum lipids and coagulation factors in healthy postmenopausal women. JAMA 279:1445

Weiner CP, Lizasoain I, Baylis SA et al. (1994) Induction of calcium-dependent nitric oxide synthases by sex hormones. Proc Natl Acad Sci USA 91:5212–5216

Wenger NK, Speroff L, Packard B (1993) Cardiovascular health and disease in women. N Engl J Med 329:247–526

Wenger NK, Knatterud GL, Canner PL (2000) Early risks of hormone therapy in patients with coronary heart disease. J Am Med Assoc 284:41–43

WHI (Women's Health Initiative) HRT Update. Available at:
http://www.nhlbi.nih.gov/whi/HRTUpdate2001.pdf

References

Williams JK, Adams MR, Herrington DM, Clarkson TB (1992) Short-term administration of estrogen and vascular responses of atherosclerotic coronary arteries. J Am Coll Cardiol 20:452–457

Wilson PWF, Garrison RJ, Castelli WP (1985) Postmenopausal estrogen use, cigarette smoking, and cardiovascular morbidity in women over 50: the Framingham Study. N Engl J Med 313:1038–1043

Writing Group for the Women's Health Initiative Investigators (2002) Risks and benefits of estrogen plus progestin in healthy postmenopausal women. Principal results from the Women's Health Initiative Randomized Controlled Trial. J Am Med Assoc 288:321–333

Future Directions

References **209**

For decades coronary heart disease (CHD) has incorrectly been viewed as being insignificant in female morbidity and mortality. There are two reasons for this:

1. In the past, most clinical trials were conducted in patients between 40 and 70 years of age. For this age group, the incidence of CHD is indeed higher in men than in women, but this disregards the fact that the incidence in women approximates that in men after age 70 years.
2. The Framingham study demonstrated that angina in women is associated with a relatively good prognosis; however, the Framingham study was likewise almost exclusively limited to middle-aged women. There is also the fact that angina occurs principally more frequently in women than in men, but that angina (without EKG changes, positive enzyme, or other objective findings) correlates poorly with cardiovascular mortality.

The fact is, CHD is *the* leading cause of death in women. Thirty percent of all female deaths are attributable to CHD. Indeed, a further increase can be expected with life expectancy generally on the rise. Despite a gradual rethinking, more than 50 % of all women in the twenty-first century still believe that cancer – and above all breast cancer – represents the greatest threat to their health and tops mortality statistics. In reality, however, twice as many women die from CHD as from cancer. Only 1 of 9 women die from breast cancer but 1 of 2 women from cardiovascular disease.

There is good reason to believe that in the future CHD will be perceived as a health problem of women. Only then will suitable prevention, early diagnosis, and timely therapy be possible, and only then will it be possible to achieve a reduction in morbidity and mortality. As long as women – and physicians – are not aware that CHD represents a health threat to women that needs to be taken seriously, women will continue to postpone office visits for "cardiac" complaints, and physicians will either consider angina to be harmless or not recognize it as such. The ultimate consequences of delayed diagnosis and therapy are a reduction in the quality of life and in life expectancy.

Regardless of gender, prevention has the greatest impact on reduction in morbidity and mortality of a disease. Aside from early diagnosis and treatment of risk factors, early and non-invasive diagnosis of CHD is desirable. Procedures such as electron-beam computed tomography and magnetic resonance tomography are certainly a first step in this direction but are not yet sufficiently refined to recognize non-calcified atherosclerotic plaques, on one hand, or the severity and/or vulnerability of stenosis, on the other. In the foreseeable future it will probably be possible to differentiate arteriosclerotic coronary arteries from normal ones with non-invasive techniques and further differentiate stable plaques from unstable ones, and hence differentiate high-risk from low-risk patients. Early recognition and treatment of vulnerable plaques would not only have a tremendous impact on the incidence of acute myocardial infarction, but also on the long-term outcome of women and men, and thus an essential impact on economics and health care politics as well.

Over the past decade there has been a tremendous progress in percutaneous coronary interventions, not only with respect to technical advances but also in the development of adjunctive medical therapy. Consequently, the number of procedures (and indications as well) has steadily increased. For example, the size of catheters used became increasingly smaller, and highly flexible balloons and stents with a very low profile are available. Women were, and continue to be, the primary beneficiaries of these technical improvements, since on average women have coronary vessels of smaller caliber than men and experience more frequent vascular complications. Further technical advances can be expected in the future that will make low-risk invasive therapy possible in older (and often smaller and frail) women.

None of the randomized, secondary preventive trials with estrogen, or the combination of estrogen with progesterone, have fulfilled the positive expectations associated with them. Despite the theoretically conceivable cardioprotective effect seen in numerous observational trials, thromboembolic events occur more frequently and the incidence of myocardial infarction is increased. The underlying mechanisms are most likely prothrombotic and proinflammatory effects of progestins (and potentially estrogen as well) which outweigh any effects of estrogens on atherogenesis and vasomotor function. In addition, the risk of breast cancer and possibly ovarian cancer is increased with prolonged hormone intake. Whether or not primary prevention with *estrogen alone* will reduce the risk of coronary artery disease has to be determined, but preliminary results are disappointing. Most likely hormone and estrogen replacement therapy will not be used in the future for primary and secondary prevention of CHD.

Statins, which presumably possess plaque-stabilizing and anti-inflammatory properties independent of their lipid-reducing effect, are highly likely to gain favor, particularly since inflammation appears to play a greater role in the pathogenesis of acute coronary syndromes and myocardial infarction in women than in men. This assumption is supported by the observation that women receive more benefit from statin therapy in secondary prevention than men (Sacks et al. 1996). Postmenopausal symptoms of estrogen deficiency, such as hot flashes, may be treated with serotonin reuptake inhibitors.

Women have a lower incidence of sudden cardiac death than men, a lower incidence of idiopathic atrial fibrillation, and a lower (dependent on the hormonal cycle) incidence of paroxysmal supraventricular tachycardia (Rubart and von der Lohe 1998). The causes are not yet known. The lower prevalence of CHD in young and middle-aged women may play a role, in particular the lower incidence of sudden cardiac death; however, differences in the electrophysiological properties of the heart, possibly as the result of long-term estrogen effects, may be operative as well. For example, basic research data demonstrated that the density of cardiac calcium channels is regulated by the number of estrogen receptors and hence indirectly via estrogen levels. During times of relative estrogen deficiency (e.g., in menopause), there is a high density of L-type calcium ion channels, which is associated with prolonged repolarization of ventricular myocytes, and thus potentially also with an increased occurrence of arrhythmias (Johnson et al. 1997). Moreover, estrogen-dependent alterations of the autonomic nervous system appear to have an impact on gender-based differences in the occurrence of arrhythmias. For example, estrogen elevates basal nitric oxide production, which in turn leads to inhibition of sympathetic and stimulation of vagal neurotransmitters (Elvan et al. 1997). This mechanism is potentially responsible for the cycle-dependent prevalence of paroxysmal supraventricular tachycardias in pre-menopausal women (Rosano et al. 1996). Research of gender differences in cardiac arrhythmias and their possible influence via hormones is still at a very early stage and little is known for certain. It is hoped that in the near future the combination of basic research and clinical trials will allow further insights and therapeutic starting points into this complex area.

References

Blumenthal RS, Zacur HA, Reis SE, Post WS (2000) Beyond the null hypothesis – Do the HERS results disprove the estrogen/coronary heart disease hypothesis? Am J Cardiol 85:1015–1017

Daly E, Vessey MP, Hawkins MM et al. (1996) Risk of venous thromboembolism in users of hormone replacement therapy. Lancet 348:977

Elvan A, Rubart M, Zipes DP (1997) NO modulates autonomic effects on sinus discharge rate and AV-nodal conduction in open-chest dogs. Am J Physiol 272:H263–H271

Grady D, Wenger NK, Herrington D et al. (2000) Postmenopausal hormone therapy increases risk for venous thrombembolic disease. The Heart and Estrogen/progestin Replacement Study. Ann Intern Med 132:689–696

Johnson BD, Zheng W, Korac KS et al. (1997) Increased expression of the cardiac L type calcium channel in estrogen receptor-deficient mice. J Gen Physiol 110:135–140

Mendelsohn ME, Karas RH (1999) The protective effects of estrogen on the cardiovascular system. N Engl J Med 340:1801

Ridker PM, Hennekens CN, Rifai N et al. (1999) Hormone replacement therapy and increased plasma concentration of C-reactive protein. Circulation 100:713

Rosano GM, Leonardo F, Sarrel PM et al. (1996) Cyclical variation in paroxysmal supraventricular tachycardia in women. Lancet 347:786–788

Rubart M, von der Lohe E (1998) Sex steroids and cardiac arrhythmia: More questions than answers. J Cardiovasc Electrophyiol 9:665–667

Sacks FM, Pfeffer MA, Moye et al. (1996) The effect of pravastatin on coronary events after myocardial infarction in patients with average cholesterol levels. N Engl J Med 335:1001–1009

Weiner CP, Lizasoain I, Baylis SA et al. (1994) Induction of calcium-dependent nitric oxide synthases by sex hormones. Proc Natl Acad Sci U S A 91:5212–5216